Colour Blindness – The Unwritten Code
By
Naomi Davies

A Parent's Guide to Colour Blindness
What to do if your child is Colour Blind

Note: The UK English spelling of Colour is used throughout the text of this book.

All pictures and photos used are copyright free. When viewing any referenced computer sites, be aware that there may be some colour distortions or differences on some screens.

Dedication

This book is lovingly dedicated to my family. Thanks to my parents who taught me so much about colour and are responsible for my early understanding of colour blindness. Also to my brother who never teased my about my *'special'* view of colour.

To my husband who is my soul mate, my constant companion and interpreter of colour. Thank you for all your help and encouragement in writing this book.

To my daughter who is my *'style guru'* and willing companion in all my shopping escapades.

To my son who never lets his colour vision limit his world.

Also to dear friends Chris and Geoff, Reg and Margaret, who have supported us with great encouragement and proof reading skills.

Contents

Who discovered colour blindness?
Are there different types of colour blindness?
Are women better with colours than men?
How or when do you test for colour blindness? As a toddler, child or adult.
Does colour affect our everyday choices?
What is the importance of colour?
How can we help people in their everyday life who are colour blind?
What does a colour blind person see?
What is a cone?
What is a rod?
Where are cones and rods found?
Do people dream in colour?
Does the colour of our eyes affect colour blindness?

Chapter 8 - Conclusions

Appendix – Colour Vision and Animals

How do we test animals for colour blindness?
Do animals see the same as humans?
Can animals be colour blind?

Resources

Chapter 1 - Introduction

This book is written primarily for parents who discover their child is colour blind. It is written to take the mystery out of colour blindness. If you have just discovered your child is colour blind then I have some really good news for you. Colour blindness need not hamper your child's development.

- Your child will still grow up like other children.
- They will have dreams of what they want to be when they are older.
- They will grow up to adulthood even though they are colour blind.
- You will have good days and bad days in parenting like everyone else.
- They will still have good friends as they grow up.
- They will mature and get married and have children like everyone else.

I have written this book to show you that your child can still achieve great things. Colour blind people become leaders of their country, great athletes, and can have a very successful life. This book is written to help you to equip your child to reach their full potential. You will find that being colour blind is not the end of the world. It can be a much more positive thing in your family life, as well as setting your child on the path for a successful future.

Throughout my life, I have been aware of an *'unwritten code'*. This coded message is written in colour and those of us, who cannot see it, need to find other means of discovering its messages. People with full colour vision do not give this code a second thought and instinctively follow it as it aids them through their everyday life. Those of us who are colour blind still need to learn it.

I hope through this book to help parents unlock this *'unwritten code'* and so enable their colour blind son or daughter to live their lives to the full in this colour coded world.

Chapter 2 - My Own Story of Discovering I Am Colour Blind

Colour blindness is something that I know a lot about because I am colour blind myself. Colour blindness runs in my family. My father was colour blind and my son is colour blind. Many people still think that girls can't be colour blind but I am living proof that both males and females can be colour blind.

I still remember the shock and disbelief that my parents had when I was very young. I was their first born and they had no expectation that I would be born with this *'problem'*, as they then saw it. I also remember the lack of knowledge and information that was available to my parents as they wrestled with the reality that I was colour blind.

In those days there was no internet. There were no general computers for everyone to use. It was the early 1950s – there was no Google. There was no simple way to find answers to my parents' questions. All the information was held in books and in the minds of medical experts. These experts were not easily accessible.

However, my father was a resourceful man. He and my mother needed answers. You see, my father already knew the reality of colour blindness as he himself was colour blind. However, it didn't explain why I was colour blind, because I was a girl and girls couldn't be colour blind – or could they?

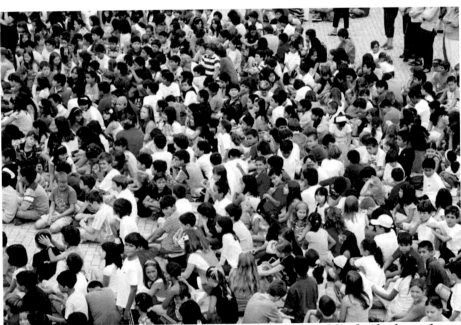

There are about 7% of boys and 0.4% of girls who are colour blind. The law of averages dictates that there will be children in this picture above who are colour blind!

I also remember that first visit, when I was in Junior School, to the *'specialist'*. This was to give my parents the results that I was *'Officially Colour Blind'*. My parents obviously already knew I had problems with colours, and was in fact colour blind. They had always made me feel that it was just one of those things that can happen and not a more major problem, like actually being blind. It was just a part of my life that we had to manage.

My father went with me to the appointment. My parents thought that, as he knew more about it, he would find it easier to understand any comments made and advice given at the meeting. They wanted to make sure I understood everything. Unfortunately, the dear lady who was tasked to break the news to us spoke in hushed tones. She even tried to silence my father when he spoke about it in such a normal way. For the first time I felt there was something wrong with me and that I had a problem. I was defective!

My father spent his whole life asking questions, he was an intelligent man who liked to understand things. He had to know why I was colour blind. I will share his discoveries and those I have made through my own life experience. Over the years I have met many people who have had lots of questions about colour blindness. This has led me to do my own research, much of which I am sharing through this book.

Even now I find some commentators on the television doing the *'science'* bit and still saying that girls cannot be colour blind! It has dawned on me that there may be others who suddenly find that their son or daughter is colour blind and it is a surprise, and perhaps a shock to them. After the shock comes the guilt, which is completely misplaced as our genetic make-up is not something we should feel guilty about. Genetics make us who we are but do not define us. Indeed there is still much that is not generally known about this topic.

My aim is to help parents understand the nature of colour blindness. It also includes ways in which parents can guide their child to work through the reality of living in a colour coded society. Those of us who are colour blind need to understand the benefits, as well as the pitfalls, of being colour blind. Family and friends need to understand too, as understanding brings freedom and appreciation for everyone.

- Both boys and girls can be colour blind.
- There are tests that can confirm colour blindness.
- Not all experts know all the answers about colour blindness.
- Colour blindness is genetically inherited.
- We should not feel guilty about our genetic make-up.
- We can equip our children to live life to the full.
- Genetics may determine who or what we are, but they need not define us.
- It is helpful if family, friends and schools understand colour blindness.

Chapter 3 - A Short History of Colour Blindness

Historically, we trace our knowledge of colour blindness from a man called John Dalton. He was a chemist born in 1766 who, along with his brother, was colour blind. His first scientific paper was entitled *'Extraordinary facts relating to the vision of colours'* and published in 1793.

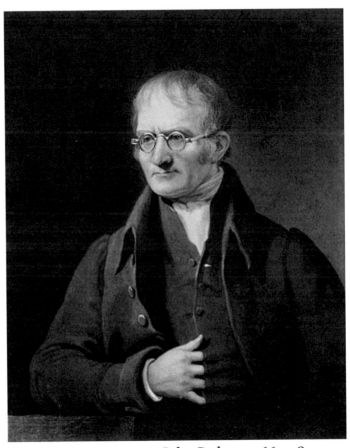

John Dalton 1766 - 1844

Both he and his brother were colour blind with the red and green colour bar. As a result of his early work, colour blindness is sometimes referred to as Daltonism. When he died from a stroke, he donated his eyes to research. He thought that the colour of the fluid in the eyeball was the cause of the problem. The picture below shows a diagram of a human eye. The liquid he was referring to is known as *'vitreous'* and is shown in the *'vitreous chamber'*. As you can see, it fills up quite a big proportion of the eye.

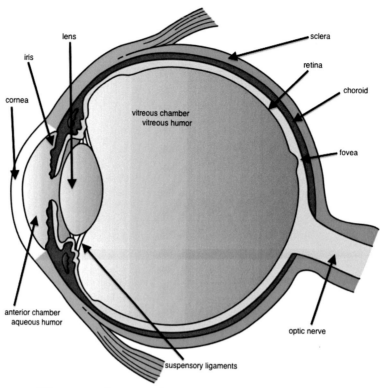

Diagram of an eye showing the liquid in the eye.

Further testing by other scientists after his death proved that this was not the case and that the *'vitreous'* liquid did not affect our colour vision. As a result of his selfless act, much has been discovered about colour blindness. It was realised that the problem must lie in the area of some deficiency in the sensory power of the eye or brain.

Before John Dalton, Isaac Newton had worked on this topic too. He discovered about the different hues of colour the eye can see coupled with the impact of different light levels. Later I am sure that John Logie Baird used much of the existing research too in his early work on televisions. Indeed, all this work has led to the creation of films in *'Technicolor'*, colour television, computers and transmitted colour, overhead projectors, and many more things that we take for granted.

For me one of the most amazing things to realise is that colour is our own interpretation of light waves. Our eyes see the light waves and our brains translate these as colour. The rainbow seen in the sky after a storm is perhaps one of the most stunning examples of colour as seen through light waves.

- John Dalton was a renowned scientist, regarded as one of the most important pioneers of colour blindness
- He and his brother were colour blind.
- Colour blindness is also called *'Daltonism'*
- Scientific work on colour led to use of colour in films, television, computers, etc.
- Colour is how our brains interpret what our eyes see as light waves – like a rainbow.

Chapter 4 - Colour Blindness

What is colour blindness?

To answer this question we must first briefly consider colour itself. In the previous chapter on *'A short history of colour blindness'*, we learnt that colour is not something that is really permanent, as it can change the way it appears in different types of light. Using the analogy of a rainbow as mentioned in Chapter 3, we can show that colour is visually perceived. It is not a solid fixed thing.

This makes it really hard to explain in layman's terms but, colour is actually light! Look at the picture of the rainbow below and you will start to see the point that I am making about the way in which light causes colour to change. Light refraction through rain is a perfect example of this phenomenon.

Our eyes are very special and, as any student of biology will know, they are our window to the world. Through our eyes we see shapes and objects that we learn to call mum, dad, brother, sister, aunty, uncle, grandmother, grandfather, trees, flowers, teddy, ball, and so on.

We also perceive light and dark and how some things sparkle in the light. However there is more to our sight than shapes and sizes.

It is generally thought that colour is perceived by humans in categories known as red, green, blue, and others. Indeed colour comes from the effects of light hitting different surfaces. This explains how things can look like one colour in one light, and another tone/shade/colour in another light.

As I said earlier, perhaps the best illustration I can give is the rainbow that comes in the sky (usually after a downpour of rain when the sun is still shining). This illustrates how colours can have different depths and intensities. How they can run from one shade or colour into another.

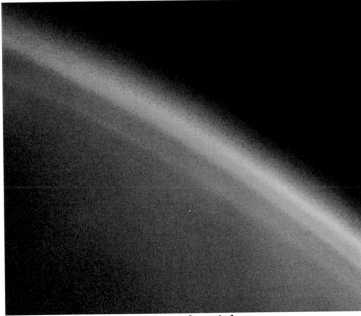

A picture of a rainbow

Indeed the rainbow is to me a perfect example of how light waves can be perceived as colour, just as sound waves we hear, can be interpreted as different noises e.g. speech, a car door slamming, the sound of footsteps, running water, etc.

The science of colour is sometimes called *'chromatics'*. It considers the way colour is *'seen'* by our human eyes and how our brain interprets that information. We learn from physics about *'electromagnetic radiation'* in ranges that we can see or in other words *'light'*.

There are many eminent scientists who have studied this at great length. From as far back as Aristotle, Sir Isaac Newton and many others through to the present day, they have wrestled with colour and how best to explain it.

They liken colour to be seen by us as light waves that we see in different strengths, depending on the time of day and the surroundings of where we are at the time. We could be on a mountain top, in a darkened room, shining a torch, etc. Everything around us can affect our perception of what we see.

The science of light

The diagram below shows some of the light wave lengths that are recorded as colour by scientists.

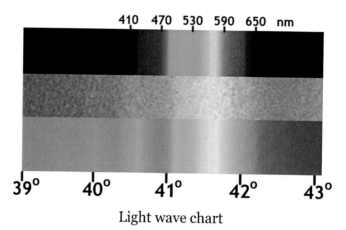

Light wave chart

As a result of their work we now have coloured lights, television, internet usage, paints, dyes for clothes, the discovery of basic palettes of colour and the knowledge of how we can make different colours. The reality of this makes me look at paintings done by old masters in quite a different way. I am starting to realises how they must have spent time understanding how light would affect their finished work. To say nothing of how they learnt to create their colours!

My intention however is not to produce a science paper on colour. There are plenty of books and other resources that are far more knowledgeable. They also go into much greater depth than I am able. My intention is to explain enough about what colour is, to help understand its impact on all our lives, and to understand what we see when we open our eyes.

- Colour is refracted light
- The science of colour is known as *'chromatics'*
- Colour changes when it gets darker or lighter
- Colour is affected by temperature
- Old masters painted pictures while understanding how light would affect their finished work
- Colour has a significant impact on our lives

How do we see colour?

Our ability to see colour is now known to be due to the presence of receptive cells at the back of the retina in the eye. These receptors are known to respond to the actual wave lengths of the light around us, and this enables us to see colours. There are two different receptors and they are known as Cones and Rods. Firstly let us look at the receptor known as a Cone.

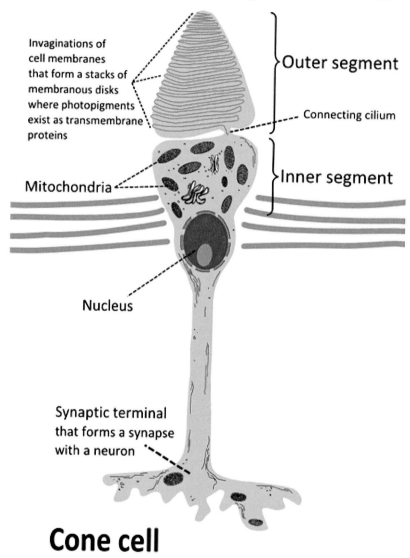

Invaginations of cell membranes that form a stacks of membranous disks where photopigments exist as transmembrane proteins

Outer segment

Connecting cilium

Inner segment

Mitochondria

Nucleus

Synaptic terminal that forms a synapse with a neuron

Cone cell

Usually, there are three types of cone cells in the eye, which in turn send different messages to the brain. One is known to respond to a violet range of colour which is known as S or short wave frequency, and sometimes called the *blue cone*. The other two are more closely connected both genetically and chemically. They are concerned with the medium and long wave colour frequencies. The M (medium) cone (also known as the *green cone*) picks up green while the L (long) cone (also called the *red cone*) perceives greenish yellow.

The diagram below shows the range of light waves that they pick up and send to our brains.

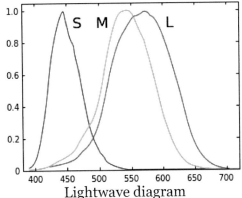

Lightwave diagram

Simply put, these three types of cone are used by our brains to interpret all the colours that we see around us.

Now let us consider the second receptor in our eyes called a rod.

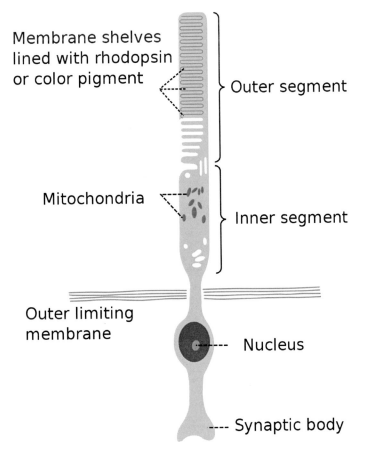

Rod Cell

The rod is a different type of receptor and is responsible for our perception of temperature.

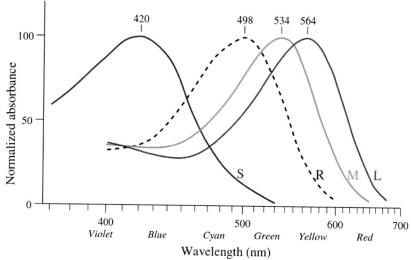

Unlike the cones (which seem to respond to light as wavelengths), the rods perceive temperature and intensity of colour, hence our ability to perceive cold and warm colours.

Here are a few examples of how differently we can see colour banks, depending on the information our brain receives from our rods and cones.

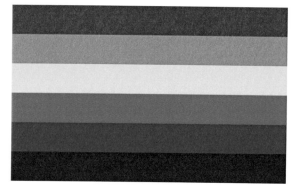

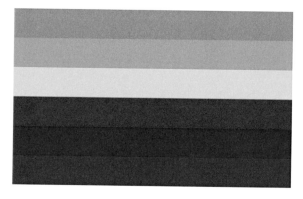

This is a set of colours as most people see them.

This is an example of how a colour blind person affected by the red/green range might see the same colours.

- Cones and rods are different receptors found in the retina of our eyes
- The 'S' cones (also known as the 'blue cones') see short wave lengths of light from the blue spectrum
- The 'M' cones (also known as 'green cones') see medium wave lengths of light from the green spectrum
- The 'L' cones(also known as the 'red cones') see long wave lengths of light, although it perceives greenish yellow
- The rods see temperature as well as the intensity of colour. They enable us to see both warm and cold colours

What causes colour blindness?

Colour blindness occurs when the colour receptors in the eye are not present or not working as they were designed to function.

As explained in the previous section, our cones help us to distinguish different wave lengths of light. John Logie Baird and others used this information to invent the television and enable us to see movies and all transmitted colour. People who are colour blind either do not have one or more of these receptors or have them but they do not function properly. While this doesn't mean we are blind to everything, it does mean we have difficulty in discerning colours.

There are different receptors in the eye which govern different aspects of colour. The way our brains interpret this information affects how we see colours. If only one receptor is malfunctioning or not present, then only one range of light wave length is affected. Hence some people have trouble with blue colours, while others have trouble with greens and reds, etc. It is dependent on which receptors are absent or malfunctioning, as to what degree of colour blindness a person experiences.

Sometimes, our receptors can become damaged through accidents or affected by drugs or by bright lights. These situations can be temporary, but sometimes they can be more permanent. My father remembered drops being put in his eyes once and he found all the colours he could see were heightened like in *'Technicolor'*.

I think it is important to mention here that it is difficult to explain colour blindness and what people actually see. This is why I find it easier to talk of light wave lengths. Many people, on first learning that I am colour blind, feel the need to ask what colour I can see. The difficulty here is that it is very hard to describe a colour, without referring to a colour for reference. For example, how do you describe the redness of red without using a colour term like crimson or scarlet, or saying it is a deeper shade of ...?

Again, I thank my father for his insight. Between us we talked about colour and my mum used her colour vision to help too. In the end, we decided that it was the depths of the colours that we perhaps didn't see. You see, both my dad and I saw the colour red, but sometimes we could confuse it with green or brown! We both enjoyed television and watching movies, so we could obviously see colour. It is worth mentioning here that there are some people who only see in monochrome i.e. black and white (or shades of grey)! The closest example of what they see is like watching the old black and white television.

Perhaps now you can understand why I prefer to talk of light wave lengths and receptors. Just as with right handedness and left handedness some people can be ambidextrous. Even our fingers have different levels of strength. In the same way, there are numerous permutations of our eyesight and colour perception. So one person who has a red/green affected view, might see a red rose slightly different to another person with a similar red/green view. An interesting fact is that in some situations any soldiers who are colour blind, may well see things that are camouflaged that their colleagues cannot see. It is useful to have such folk in your company!

There are even some people who can see pastel shades better with one eye and warm or cold colours with another eye. This and the varying abilities of colour perception, can explain why one person can match colours well and another maybe not so well. Also differences in light may explain why one person can carry a colour in their head and another not remember a shade as well, unless what they are matching is in the same room. This is especially evident when decorating and trying to remember a paint colour, or matching blinds or curtains, or even bedding and furniture.

How many couples have you heard discussing which colour or sample is best suited to their decorating needs? How many conversations have you had about which paint looks best on which wall? Over the years, more and more of us ask for samples to take home and put in the room we are decorating. Even then we need to see it at night-time as well as in the day-time. However we can still get caught with a wall paper that appears to change colour, or reveal a different pattern or tone in a different room or even on a different wall.

My husband is very accommodating of my colour vision. He tries to choose from a palette of colours that I like, so that at the end of the day we are both relaxed in the room. However, I would always defer to his colour choices, as colour and how it matches with other things in a room, is very important to him.

Indeed it is interesting to note that animals and insects see things differently to humans. This is why hunters use camouflage when seeking to catch animals and animal watchers use hides when they want to observe birds and other animals. Even the fly sees things differently to us, which explains in part why its reactions are so fast when anyone tries to swat one of them.

- Colour blindness usually happens when any of the cones or rods are malfunctioning or missing. This is generally a permanent reality.
- Colour blindness can be caused by bright lights, reaction to drugs, illness. This is generally temporary and full colour vision usually returns in time.
- There is one type of colour blindness called *monochrome* where only black and white or shades of grey are visible.
- It is hard to describe what a colour blind person sees, since colour is hard to describe without using colour as a reference.
- Many people find it difficult to carry colours in their heads when matching paints, etc. as different light settings affects how we see or remember shades of colour.
- Colour blind people appreciate different aspects of colour, but they still have their own likes and dislikes of colours.

Naomi Davies

Why are only some people colour blind, and others not colour blind?

This is a question my parents had to deal with when I was born. At first, it was not obvious that I was colour blind. In fact, it is quite hard to be certain, especially with a first born child. When my own daughter was born, it took a while for us to be certain that she wasn't affected, although we knew that because my husband wasn't colour blind she shouldn't be affected. When our son was born, we knew quite quickly and could see evidence in his colour choices.

As for how people become colour blind, I owed my first understanding to my father. He knew from school days that he had a problem with colours, but it was not until later that the term *'colour blind'* was used. In those days it was said that a person was not very good with colours, without understanding the reasons or causes.

My dad found out about genetics (as many do at school nowadays). He explained to me that we inherit many abilities and differences from our parents and we all have a genetically inherited body. This means that just as our eye and hair colours are inherited, so are many other characteristics. For example, many have special abilities in music and tendencies to be good at administration and organising. Then there is our ability to socialise or our fondness for poetry, our ability to grow plants or cook food, do craft work, the list is endless. Whether we are short or tall is also determined by our genetic make-up.

In simple terms, colour blindness, like all inherited things, is passed via our parents genes from one generation to another by chromosomes. If you were a girl then you had an XX mixture and if a boy then you had an XY mixture. Colour blindness is passed on with an X chromosome.

He showed me that for him to be colour blind, then one of his mum's X chromosomes must have had the colour blindness gene attached to it. As he only had one X chromosome he was bound to be colour blind if he inherited the X chromosome that carried the colour blindness. This meant that he could not pass it to a boy, but any daughter he had would carry this particular gene.

However, this did not explain how I was colour blind. Since my mother wasn't colour blind I surely should only carry this particular gene (or so I thought).

Then my father told me that my mother had obviously carried an X chromosome with the colour blindness too (in fact they remembered a relative on my mother's side who had had unusual colour ideas).

Finally, my father explained that, for a girl to be colour blind, she had to inherit the X from her mother that carried colour blindness as well as one from her father who would be colour blind. Then I understood that I was one of those rare people who had received two X chromosomes, both with the colour blind gene attached. Incidentally, my younger brother was not colour blind. This was because he received the X chromosome from my mum that did not have the colour blindness gene attached to it, along with the Y chromosome from my dad which does not carry this particular gene.

I know that the question of how we can inherit colour blindness is complicated. It is not easy to fully understand how things pass from one generation to another generation. Although I want to keep things simple, this aspect of inheritance is important to understand. My mother felt guilty about passing this to me, until my father explained how genetics work. When she understood that everything about who we are is passed on in this way, she realised that she was not in any way at fault.

I feel that understanding this aspect of genetic inheritance is quite important and as such is at the core of my book. In the next chapter, entitled *'Genetic Inheritance'*, I have used diagrams to show pictorially how colour blindness is passed from one generation to another generation. It also shows how one person (or sibling) can be colour blind while another is unaffected. The diagrams reveal how colour blindness can *'hide'* in a family line until it seems to unexpectedly appear, even in families where no immediate member may be known to be affected by colour blindness.

- Not all siblings in a family are colour blind.
- Girls and boys can be colour blind.
- Colour blindness is passed on by an affected X Chromosome.
- Many of our natural abilities are passed on to us via genetics.
- The way we look is determined by our genetic inheritance.

Chapter 5 - Genetic Inheritance as it relates to colour blindness

Each of the following six diagrams shows a father and a mother and the four genetic possibilities of inheritance for any child born. In other words, every time a child is born there are four possible options for their chromosome make-up.

Each child can inherit a combination of an X and a Y chromosome from their parents that decree if they will be a boy or a girl. Then there is an option of which of the two X chromosomes of the mother, goes with which X or Y chromosome from the father. The following diagram shows the inheritance chain without colour blindness being anywhere in the family.

Diagram G1

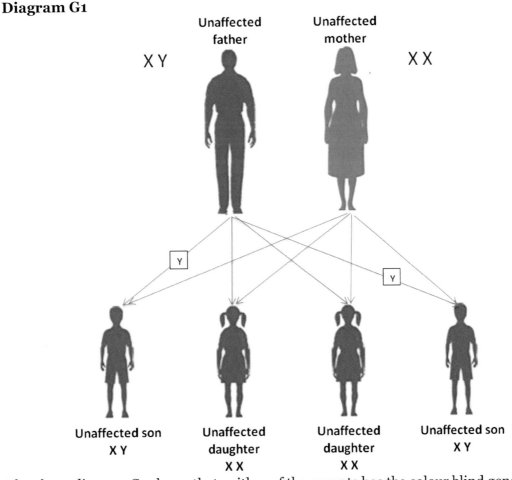

The above diagram G1 shows that neither of the parents has the colour blind gene and I have shown them in blue. So you can see that the thin arrows show how the X and Y from the parents pass to their children. This arrangement shows that firstly they either have a boy or girl, then that the parents pass their X chromosomes to their children.

So, all the above people are unaffected by colour blindness. They do not even carry an affected X chromosome. They will therefore have normal colour vision.

I will now show you how colour blindness passed through my family to show how it can be inherited. The addition of brown is to show pictorially how it is passed. So anyone coloured in brown is colour blind. Anyone coloured in blue has normal colour vision. Those who are brown and blue carry colour blindness but have normal vision. The use of X_1 is to denote the X chromosome that carries the colour blindness. I have also thickened the blue line that denotes the passing of the affected X_1 chromosome.

In the picture G2 below, you can see that my father (who was colour blind and is shown in brown) married my mother who was not colour bind. They expected that neither I, nor my younger brother, would be colour blind. My dad realised that I would carry the colour blindness from the inheritance of his X_1 chromosome, but I was not expected to be colour blind.

Diagram G2

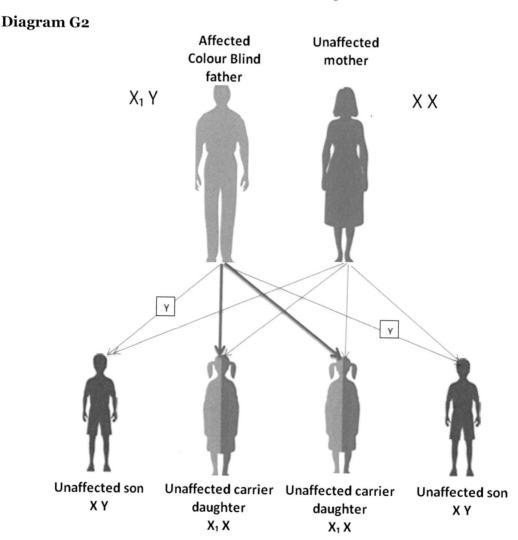

The above chart shows what they expected to happen. However, I was born colour blind. How could this be the case? The above diagram shows the thick lines for the X_1 chromosome which were passed from him to any possible combination his daughter might have and how he cannot pass it to a boy (since the boy would receive his Y chromosome which does not carry colour blindness).

My dad then explained to me the genetic option in the next diagram, which I have called G3. This shows that the only way for me to be colour blind, was if my mother was carrying the affected gene. She must therefore have a genetic make-up of $X_1 X$ (or $X X_1$).

Diagram G3

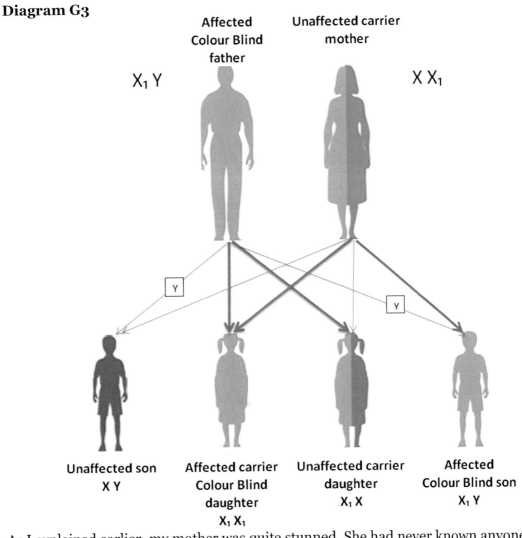

Affected Colour Blind father

$X_1 Y$

Unaffected carrier mother

$X X_1$

Unaffected son
$X Y$

Affected carrier Colour Blind daughter
$X_1 X_1$

Unaffected carrier daughter
$X_1 X$

Affected Colour Blind son
$X_1 Y$

As I explained earlier, my mother was quite stunned. She had never known anyone in her family to be colour blind. The only thing she could think of was that one of her brothers had not been good with colours. This was obviously the explanation. Neither of her parents was colour blind, so her mother must have carried it unknowingly.

As you can see from the options above, even my brother could have been colour blind. However, he inherited the clear X from my mum and so has not inherited colour blindness from our family genetic make-up. Since I inherited both the affected X_1 from my father as well as the affected X_1 from my mother, I was the one who was colour blind!

It is worth noting that while about 7% of boys are born colour blind, only 0.4% of girls are colour blind. So this is a very rare case, but not impossible.

This following picture G4, shows how the genetic inheritance continued when I married my husband.

Diagram G4

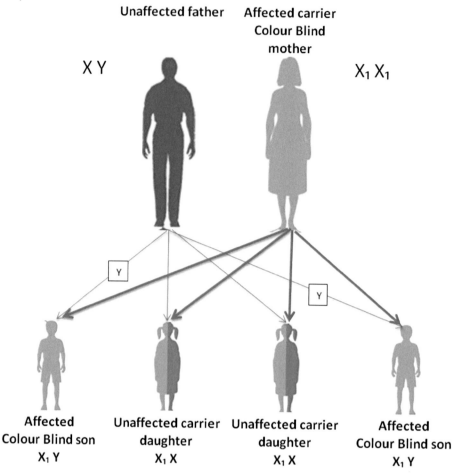

My husband is not colour blind. As you can see from this diagram any son we had, would be colour blind as is shown by the thick blue lines. This was because I could only pass on an affected X chromosome (shown as X_1). Similarly, any daughter would not be colour blind as she could only carry the affected X_1. The reason she would not be colour blind is that the X_1 denoting colour blindness is recessive. This means that her unaffected X would over-ride the affected X_1. In other words, her brain would only refer to the clear X for its colour information. She is therefore shown as half brown and half blue.

If she then marries an unaffected husband then her family will follow the same genetic path as shown in G5 below.

Diagram G5

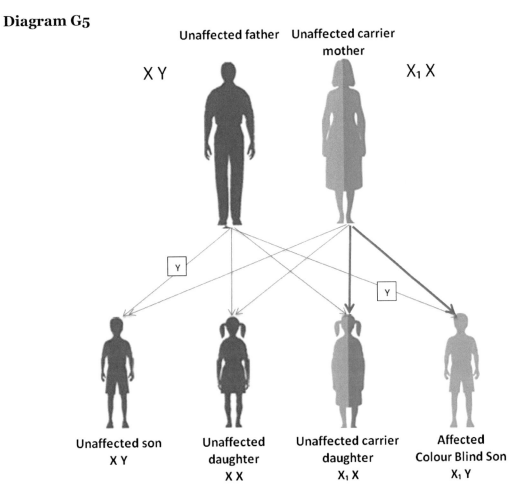

Unaffected father   Unaffected carrier mother

$X\,Y$ $X_1\,X$

Y

Y

Unaffected son
$X\,Y$

Unaffected daughter
$X\,X$

Unaffected carrier daughter
$X_1\,X$

Affected
Colour Blind Son
$X_1\,Y$

As you can see, she may or may not have a son with colour blindness. Her daughter may carry it or she may not carry it. It all depends on whether her daughter inherits the X or the X_1. This permutation occurs every time a child is born. The X or X_1 is available every time a child is conceived. Just as a child may be a boy or a girl when conceived, so the child may inherit any of the X chromosomes available. In other words they are not marked as used or cancelled but freshly available every time.

If, however, her husband were to be colour blind, then she would follow the G3 diagram above on page 23, like my parents.

This final diagram shows the last possible combination. It is when a colour blind man marries a colour blind woman. As you can see, all or any children born will be colour blind. As there are only affected X_1 chromosomes available, they are the only ones that can be passed on to the children.

Diagram G6

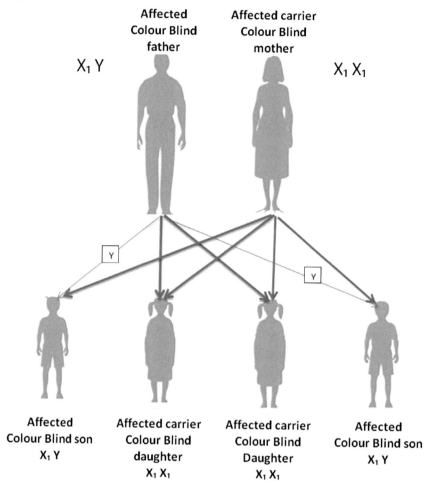

I had a lot to process in growing up. I knew it was rare for a girl to be colour blind, but at least my dad could see the world as I saw it since we had the same colour bar. In other words, we saw colours in the same way as each other. For me, this was very re-assuring and of great comfort.

I have now discovered some film clips that show how people see colour. They can be found on my website **www.colourblindnesstips.com** . They show how normally sighted people view a picture and how someone with a Red/Blue/Other colour difficulty see the picture. I think this is particularly helpful when understanding how a colour blind person sees the world. For parents who are not themselves colour blind, who find they have a child who is colour blind, it can help them to understand how their child sees the world. They can then understand why their child might make particular colour choices and know how best to help their son, or daughter, to cope in our multicolour world.

Obviously, as with all our senses, different people have different levels of perception. Some people have certain types of hearing that make them very musical and able to hear slight differences of tone, when playing instruments or singing. Other people have a heightened sense of touch, like sculptors. Others can train themselves in this, as with the ability to read braille. Artists see colours differently and use it to produce their great works of art.

Gardeners have a need for colour perception when planning their garden, or even knowing when a fruit is ripe for picking. Needlewomen need to know their designs are colour coordinated, or that their repairs blend in with the garment they are repairing. Cooks can know by smell if a food or dish is sweet enough, or by appearance if a food like meat is fully cooked.

We use all our senses in many spheres of our lives. Understanding how we use our senses can help us to balance any short comings in our senses, or even improve those we do have in our bodies. In other words, if your senses are weak in one area, your other senses will often be heightened and compensate for any limitations.

In the next chapter called *'Living with Colour Blindness'*, I will endeavour to show different ways that those of us who are colour blind can adapt to the colour coded messages throughout nature and in our modern world. My aim is to give pointers and ideas so that parents can reveal the *'unwritten code'* of colour to any child who may be colour blind. As soon as you start to consider these colour messages, you will start to realise the importance of helping the colour blind child through this maze of hidden information and warnings. These messages can vary from country to country and I am sure that once you start seeing them from your child's point of view, you will be able to include those that are part of your everyday environment.

- Colour blindness is inherited on the X (X_1 in the diagrams) chromosome.
- Colour blindness can be passed to a girl by a colour blind father but she generally carries it as it is a recessive gene.
- If a girl is only carrying colour blindness ($X_1 X$), she is not herself colour blind as it is a recessive gene. This means that the clear X will function and the affected X_1 will be dormant.
- A boy can only be colour blind if he inherits the X_1 chromosome from his mother.
- A girl can only be colour blind if she inherits it from both her mother and her father ($X_1 X_1$).
- About 7% of boys are born colour blind.
- About 0.4% of girls are born colour blind.
- We can learn to develop our other senses, like smell, to help us as we manage colour blindness.

Chapter 6 - Living with Colour Blindness

The reality of being colour blind.

Fortunately, colour blindness, although it has its challenges, is not life-threatening. As with many things we inherit, colour blindness is something that we can let define us in positive or negative ways. Is your glass half full or half empty? It is how we perceive the condition, that will determine how we live our lives.

I have never allowed my colour blindness to stop me being involved in anything I wanted to do. Basically, where there is a will there is usually a way.

I am from a family steeped in needlework and crafts. My grandmother's sister was one of the most prominent needlework women and quilters in her day. She and her team actually made the present from South Wales of a quilt on the occasion of the wedding of Queen Elizabeth II to Prince Phillip in the 1950s. I remember seeing my Great Aunt Mary in Blaina, South Wales in her front room with her team of ladies. They had special trestles and a table top made up, on which was fixed their latest quilt.

This quilt was created from layers of fabric and filling. It had a design drawn on it with French chalk using their own templates. All the ladies were meticulously hand stitching the design. Needless to say their work was quite beautiful. In fact the whole house was filled with cushions and furniture which had all been hand stitched by my aunt. I remember that, as a child, I felt quite in awe of it all and privileged to have been able to visit as often as I did. It was her daughter (my Aunt May) who many years later, taught me to hem when she was shortening a garment. The hemming was done in such a way as to make it invisible from the right or front visible side of the garment.

Even with all this heritage, I could have decided that needlework was not for me. Yet with a little help, I have been able to make garments, curtains, and much more. The skills of needlework can be learned like any other skill, but what I have trouble with is matching threads. This is simply fixed by having a trusted helper to pick out the right colour for me. My children still bring me garments to repair or alter, while my husband picks out the right colour.

- Colour blindness does not need to define who we become, or what we do, in life as we grow up.
- Needlework skills can still be learnt.
- Being colour blind does not mean you can't see colour, but that you may need help in matching fabric and thread colours.
- By adapting to our own vision of colour, we can do most tasks we want to do, even if we need a little help.

Colour blindness and shopping

This is a surprising topic and few people consider the impact of colour in the world of commerce. This is one of the areas when the 'unwritten code' is quite prevalent. When shopping for items, it is important to read all the labels to make sure that what you buy is the correct version of the item that you want to purchase. For example let's consider milk. It is important to be aware that not all shops use the same shade of colour for the lids of their milk and other fresh goods. I can never be sure which version I have picked up. I have to read the labels every time to make sure that I am buying fully skimmed milk and not semi or full cream, or some other product that looks as if it might be milk!

This is the same with any packaging. No matter what it looks like, I will need to read the label. This means that shopping can take me a little longer as I cannot use the colour codes to help me. Needless to say, I am a bit mystified with the colour coding that happens to denote fat content, etc. on some foods.

I also have to be careful with money. I know that often there are different size notes, but I prefer to read the markings on the paper money. This way I know if I have given a £10.00 note and not a £20.00 note, because I have actually read it.

Coins are also a constant source of confusion. The original penny pieces and other coins like the very old three-penny piece, used to be easier to distinguish by shape and thickness, as well as by size. Nowadays, one has to check that our monarch's head is on the coins to be sure that it is our currency. Then we have to read the information to be sure of its value, especially with the introduction of the newer coins. There is a lot of standardisation that can make it more difficult to tell one coin from another. This can be further complicated with the possibility of foreign coins getting into circulation by mistake.

Whenever I am in a different country this becomes even harder, as I am not so familiar with the notes. I am always checking the written words as I can never be sure of the colour. Again the coins need to be looked at carefully, so that I give the right amount when paying for things and be alert to check my change.

- Teach your child to look for signs other than colour when shopping.
- Be patient if they get it wrong.
- Colour coded packaging will not have the same impact for them as those with normal colour vision.
- Consider the coinage and notes in one's home country as well as when travelling abroad.

Colour blindness and fashion.

Just because someone is colour blind doesn't mean they cannot enjoy fashion. There may be some limitations but these should be viewed as challenges!

Colour vision does not affect our fashion sense. What clothes styles suit us can be taught or learnt, like any other skill. We can soon know what style of jacket or dress or trousers looks best on us and then we have to discover what colour looks good too.

When I was a child, my mum took time to help me choose what styles looked good and also what colours looked best on me. This was before the days of Colour Advisers! The trick is to find out what colours you like and which look good on you. We cannot dress in just what everyone else likes, we have to develop our own style and colour preferences. My mum realized that she would have to teach me a basic colour palette, as she would not always be there to tell me what colour looked best with another.

So we went for a base colour of brown and chose tops and jewellery to match. I opted for bright colours and wore pinks and deep blues and reds or cream. I would usually opt for gold coloured jewellery and brown and cream beads. This meant I had a fair chance of looking coordinated to others, while feeling good in my own choice of clothing. I admit that a whole section of my brain is used to remember colour rules like grass is green, fire engines and fire extinguishers are red, as well as that striped tee-shirt I bought last week will go with the red three quarter trousers I bought last year.

Although I now have more help available when I need advice, I freely admit that planning what I am wearing for a given occasion, or even packing clothes for a holiday, are among my most difficult tasks. The basic lessons my mum taught me when I was a child, are still the ones I use now as an adult. I have a range of colours that I use, but I also think of what looks right in nature to give me a guide. Shopping for clothes is a really good excuse for a day out with my daughter as she has become my fashion guru. She and my husband have picked up my mum's guidance. They understand that it is not just about choosing items that look good on me. It is also about them using their colour vision to choose colours that I like and can see that suit me too.

Another issue that is not often noticed is that clothes sizes are colour coded. Fortunately they also have size numbers as well, but it means that a colour blind person has to read everything and cannot use colour to quickly scan for the right size garment. It would also be so helpful if manufacturers could print the colour on more garment labels. It is happening with some items and hopefully the trend will continue.

- Colour blindness does not affect our fashion sense.
- Teach your child about colours and how they match with others. Tell them about different shades of brown so that they know what khaki is like, etc.
- Help your child to build a base wardrobe. Encourage them to have a base colour like black, brown, navy or grey and then to match shirts or blouses in white or cream, etc. for the full co-ordinated look.
- Consider a colour advisor so that they can have a palette of colours to use when they go shopping for clothes.
- You need to include colours that your colour blind child can see and like, as well as ones that suit him/her.

Colour blindness & make-up

When you are not sure of colour or depths of colour, it can be a challenge to wear make-up but not impossible. I admit that I don't wear it all the time, but I have devised my own way of using it. It is also helpful that most make-up has its colour written on it, which is invaluable information.

Generally it is best to work out a colour scheme with a trusted family member or close friend, or even a beauty make-up expert. I prefer to stick to a range of colours that I know from previous experience will go with anything I might wear. I stick to this small range of options. As with all things, one needs to experiment, but the rule is to keep it simple.

When using make-up, I would always advocate using a little to enhance the appearance, rather than using a lot to make a dramatic statement. The reality is that colour errors, or mismatched colours, are readily seen by those with normal colour vision. This will make someone stand out as an eyesore, rather than enhancing their natural beauty with the help of make-up.

I have recently experimented with the *'Liz Earl'* range of cosmetics and found it reasonably easy to use. Like all things involving colour, it is important to do it in a good light. My daughter and I had a brilliant day out visiting the *'Liz Earl'* make-up specialist in their Guildford (Surrey, UK) premises. The lady was very helpful and, with my daughter's support, came up with a relatively easy and simple range of colours and products for me to use. So whether I wanted to use make-up every day, or on a special occasion, I had something I was confident of using.

It is also important to use the colour vision you have and try to memorize shades that you can see. For example, when I apply a little blusher on my cheek bones, I look to check that it is a similar shade of depth or darkness to each cheek. Similarly with eye shadow, you get used to seeing an acceptable comparison. After a few checks with a close friend, you can gain confidence that you can look good with make-up if you want to use it. I also find a light dusting with powder on the face, or gentle blending of eye shadow helps too.

- Always keep make-up simple. Make-up is meant to enhance beauty not make you stand out like a beacon.
- Use a make-up advisor.
- Practice applying the make-up, so that you are used to the way colours look. Then you can be more confident that each eye lid matches and the colours blend, etc.

Colour blindness at work.

This can be challenging, depending on the type of job you have, but by no means impossible.

Some people never realize they are colour blind, indeed when my parents were children in the 1940s, it was not high on the agenda.

However, in today's high tech world it can be a little more daunting but, with forethought & planning, it need not be a serious problem for most professions. Even so, I once read of a man who was a rug repairer. He got into difficulties when the owner was away. He just repaired a rug as he had always done, but used the wrong colour thread. To him the job was perfect but to the customer, the colour choice made the neat repair stand out in a glaringly obvious way!

Let us consider the work in an office. If someone uses colour alone to code files and make calendar appointments, then there could be a problem. However, simply by adding shape such as red triangles, yellow circles, etc. the problems can be avoided. This means that a colour sighted person can use colour to quickly find their information and a colour blind person can find the same information by using the shape reference. We basically need to consider our work place and how we can make it user friendly for everyone, no matter what their colour vision.

One of the major problems is what happens if a colour blind person does not see colour coded messages. If they don't know they are there, then they cannot use this means of information. This means they need to be far more vigilant. For example, I am not a sailor, but I am told that boats have different coloured lights at night. This means that if I was applying for this job, I would probably fail the tests as I would find it difficult to distinguish between the different coloured lights.

Any person who guides ships or boats into harbour at night cannot do this without help. Even if you are sailing as a pleasure or hobby, it is safer to have someone with you, unless you have devised a method to compensate for your colour vision. It obviously depends on the type of colour blindness.

Colour blindness can affect all walks of life. In the building world, I know of a brick layer who when mixing 'muck' is very careful to measure everything. For example, when he needs to add dye to mortar and cement he creates the right colour mix by carefully measuring the amount of dye put in each mix with the number of same size shovels. This ratio is repeated from load to load and so the same colour mix is produced. This is what I call 'using your own gauge or shade reference' so that even if you are colour blind, you can still produce the same result.

I once knew of an electrician whose colour bar was such that he could still distinguish between the wire colours, and was passed as fit to do the job, since his colour vision did not impair his work. This illustrates the fact that not all colour bars have the same impact. After all even Beethoven found a way to continue to compose music although he was partly deaf in later years. He used the vibration of the notes as his guide in composing, along with his memory of sound, and what hearing he still had remaining.

Another example of difficult situations not being life-threatening is with driving. Traffic lights are noted for their order rather than colour.

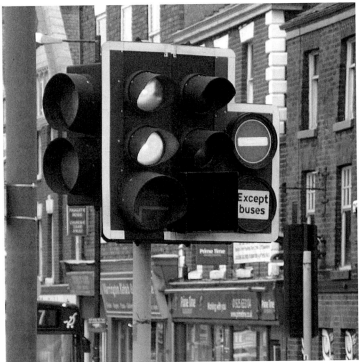

Set of traffic lights in UK.

'At the top you stop,
in the middle you get ready
and below you go'.

This was a regular rhyme at home, but it got the point home and made driving easier. However, a sign of the need for greater vigilance can be found in the fact that motorway road lights are different colours. This was something I did not know until I had been driving for many years. I could not use the colours on the road markings to help me. I just had the lights and my awareness of where everyone was to guide me. For me, knowing I am colour blind means that I am always on the lookout! I know I cannot be complacent and it makes me much more aware and alert to my surroundings. I always look for the unexpected and try to be ready for anything that might, or might not, happen. This is true for anyone in this day and age with fast moving traffic and lights everywhere.

We all have some kind of limitation or challenge. The important thing is not to let our limitations define us, but to find innovative ways to forge our own destiny. I always view my colour-blindness as a blessing, since although a very slight handicap, it enables me to empathise with others and be aware that we all have some challenges.

After all some people, as they get older, find their hearing reduces, some their eyesight, some their fitness reduces, some their mobility lessens, some become forgetful. It is not what happens to us but *'recognising'* what is happening that is important. Then it is *'how'* we deal with any resulting issues that will determine our character and the quality of life we can have. In other words, we all have challenges. Let us all look out for each other and make life easier for everyone.

- Try and use colours and symbols in diaries.
- Consider what colours are used in presentations.
- Learn the traffic lights rhyme.
- Be aware of warning signs at work.
- Always be alert to signs of danger and be aware of what is happening around you.
- Choose a career carefully and look for ways around colour if your job is impacted by it.

Colour blindness and health.

Home is a safe environment. But there are a few things to consider with regard to colour blindness. Someone who is colour blind will not always know if they or a family member become pale in the face. We cannot always see the colour change. I had to be very careful especially when my children were very young and look for other indicators if they were unwell.

Another skin change we cannot see is when someone starts to go red in the sun. We can't see any change until it has already happened. Our children were always covered in sunscreen when on holiday to protect them from getting burnt.

- When a child is ill look for other signs such a temperature.
- Get another parent or friend to check for paleness.
- Be quick to re-act if your child is unwell and faints or becomes dizzy.
- Be aware that those who are colour blind cannot recognize the early warning signs of sunburn and may not know they have caught too much sun.

Colour blindness & cooking

This is a surprising area. Firstly, yes I can cook, but I do make adjustments. For example, the recipe says cook the biscuits until they are a light fawn colour. I adjust this and look for them to have changed their shade by the time I have allowed, and take them out before they get dark. My family love eating my biscuits, so I must have got it right! I have learnt to use different gauges when cooking, including my sense of smell!

When providing family dinners, it is also important to use the timer, especially for meat. Clear juices look clear, but then I have learnt what clear looks like for me!

My father always used to say with toast, *'when it's brown it's done but when it's black it's finished'*! My dad had a great sense of humour. He and I found all sorts of ways around preparing and cooking food. One food I enjoy is bacon, but I do find it quite hard to get it just right. My dad used to let it get quite crispy as he said he liked it that way!

My husband is a great believer in timing everything. As a result, I have learnt that I can even cook steaks in a frying pan with a timer and constant turning of the meat. Perhaps that is why, although I can cook a wide variety of foods, I have always preferred to cook stir-fry meals, Shepherd's Pie and make up all sorts of interesting dishes that didn't require looking for colour changes!

When I was younger I would stick meticulously to a recipe, but as I grew in confidence I would vary things. I also used my sense of smell and would smell the sweetness and flavours of dishes as well as taste them.

- Get your child use to cooking in the kitchen.
- Be aware that old style electric rings are hard to see if they are live, especially when first turned on or on a low setting.
- Teach your child to time things when cooking.
- Cook together and enable them to learn what clear juices look like for them.
- When cooking biscuits, cake, or even toast, it is the smell as well as the shade of colour that tells us when something is cooked.
- A colour blind person appreciates how food looks and can be guided to choose different coloured ingredients so that everyone can appreciate the end result.

Colour blindness in school

This is a very interesting topic that is changing all the time. When I was at school, I tended to keep quiet about my colour blindness and only a few of my close friends knew about it. This was for a number of reasons.

Perhaps I should start at the beginning. My parents always knew that I was colour blind and to me it was a normal aspect of life. I did everything that all children did from jigsaws to painting. My parents encouraged me to try everything and helped me to develop different methods of coping. The difference was that I didn't understand it as coping, but as learning how to do things.

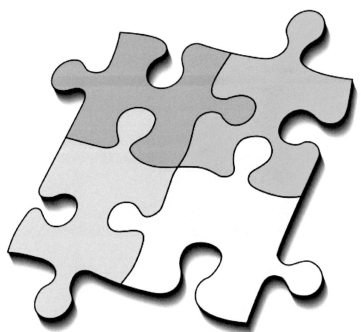

It is best to use full-interlocking jigsaws.

For example, I loved (and still do) jigsaws but colour was not always the best aid to knowing where a particular piece would go. Therefore I learnt to use shapes and developed lots of patience as I tried different pieces of sky, or grass, or tree, to work out which one would fit!

When I was at the end of my Junior School, the class did what was called colour tests and it was then that I was officially diagnosed as being colour blind. A meeting was set up at an education department in my town. My father decided it was best if he came with me as he knew a lot about colour blindness and felt he would be the best person to be with me, especially as he was colour blind too.

It was at this meeting that I came to realize that there might be a problem with being colour blind. I was very confused and I think my dad was a little angry. I don't think the dear lady officer knew much about colour blindness and, while my dad was happy to discuss it in front of me, she felt it should be discussed in hushed tones. This left me feeling odd and awkward. In fact I remember asking my dad if there was something wrong with me. He very patiently explained that this was nothing we didn't already know, and that there was nothing seriously wrong with me.

Looking back, I suppose it is like all things, if people don't understand then they don't know how to deal with it. The lady probably thought she was going to have to drop a bombshell and say that against all odds I was colour blind and would have to deal with this difficulty for my whole life. Whereas my parents had always known that I was colour blind and none of us saw it as anything insurmountable.

Nowadays, with the progress in technology and methods of teaching, it is essential for schools to know which children are colour blind. Since 7% of boys and 0.4% of girls are colour blind, there are likely to be some affected children in every school. I trained as a teacher in the early 1970s and once came upon a school that used colour to help teach mathematics. I remember some consternation when it was discovered that one of the children was colour blind and so they had to revise their methods. The sad thing is that there will have been quite a few of their young students who were also colour blind – but that was back in the 1960s.

When our own children started school, they had what was called a colour table in their Nursery Class. Each week it was a different colour and everyone had to take an item of that colour into school for the colour table. This was a novel way to teach colour, as everyone has to learn the names of different colours. It was interesting to see how many different shades of one colour there were and this added a new dimension for those who were colour blind. It also helped children with normal colour vision, to appreciate that not everyone saw the world as they did but that that was normal and part of life.

As our children progressed to senior school, it became evident that there were some scientific experiments that were harmful to colour blind children. By then we had established that our son was colour blind and so, when the teacher asked if anyone was colour blind, he put his hand up. When the teacher queried if he really was colour blind and not just having a joke, his friends confirmed that he was, since some of them had known him from Infant School, a positive benefit of others understanding!

This is another thing that is often missed. Have you ever heard someone say, *'I've done something wrong and I don't know what it is?'* If it happened in the wood work class or in a reading group, it may be that the tools or books are put away in colour coded ways, and the child has not realised that they have done anything wrong. This can happen especially if a child is born into a family with no real knowledge of colour blindness. This could mean that no one has picked up that the child is actually colour blind, and not just a bit slow to pick things up.

Even when writing on a board or using computer diagrams, it is important to consider what colours are used. This is because there are some colours that adults as well as children cannot see. Many people cannot see yellow. Some find red, green and brown hard to distinguish. Sometimes black and red can be difficult. If you start to add aquas and limes to the colour palette, you may be surprised to find that many more people will find it hard to follow. The affect for a fully colour-sighted person may be really beautiful and appealing. However, for a colour blind person it becomes almost impossible to understand what they are looking at, let alone see it properly.

Many churches are now using overheads and computer screens to make things more interesting and appealing. Unfortunately, the wrong choice of background colour can make it really hard to read the words of a hymn or chorus on the screen, let alone keep up with everyone singing!

Although many of my examples have an element of humour, there is also a feeling of frustration. This is because there appears to be an *'unwritten code'*. All around us are examples of colour coded messages that can only be picked up easily by full colour sighted children and adults. It is done so naturally by colour sighted people that they are unaware of the impact it can have on others.

One of the reasons I have written this book is to ensure that colour sighted people are aware of these hidden messages and can perhaps realise that not everyone can read them. My heart immediately goes out to those who are always in trouble but don't know why. Few people stop to think that the reading book put in the wrong pile, or the green measuring tools put on the wrong shelf, or the artwork done on the wrong colour paper, are anything other than someone being naughty.

- Encourage the use of jigsaws but make sure they are fully interlocking and that they have lots of definite detail. Jigsaws are regarded as a useful pre reading activity. It is important to look at shape as well as colours.
- Talk to your school and make them aware that your child is colour blind. Then they can make sure that any colour coding used in reading or the sorting of tools, etc. are organised so as not to exclude your son or daughter.
- If there is a colour table, help your child to participate so that they learn what colours look like for them.
- Get colouring pencils that have their colour names printed on.
- Basic, or primary, colours are easier to see than more complicated colours like aqua and lime

Colour blindness and jobs in and around the home

Colour blindness rarely affects the ability to put up pictures or shelves or even to assemble furniture units, assuming you have this handy skill. However, it can affect how you put up wallpaper and paint. It can be hard to match wallpaper patterns and their colours, so a second opinion is useful. My dad used to paint but my mum had to tell him when he missed bits. The first coat wasn't too bad but with the second coat he never knew which bits he'd done. My mum had to stand behind him and tell him which bits he had missed. In the end they decided to get a decorator in to help them.

In the garden, mowing the lawn and digging or even planting is not a problem. Weeding is not too bad either with care. However, knowing when fruit was ripe and ready to pick could be tricky. As could planning a colour theme of flowers in the garden!

Car maintenance is another consideration. My dad was a tool maker and found general maintenance was not too difficult, but he would need a friend to tell him the colour of the exhaust on an engine so that he would know if it was too rich, etc. Maybe that's why he always had a friend round to work on vehicles.

- Always have a second opinion when decorating and doing jobs involving colour in the home.
- All the above jobs seem to be best with a helper.
- When teaching children or young people to do any of these jobs, it is important to take into consideration any colour issues and to show them how best to deal with them.

- ### *Colour blindness & sewing*

If you are colour blind it doesn't mean you can't sew! It means you find colours difficult to see and match with other colours. Knowing how to do a French seam is very useful, as is sewing on a button or hemming a garment, or even how to make clothes and curtains.

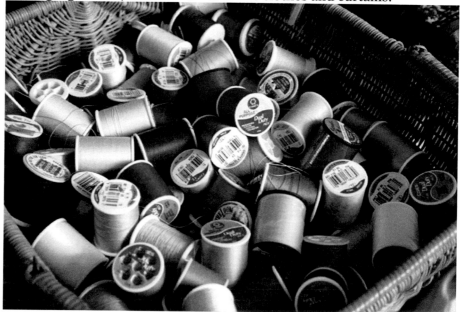

Assorted cotton reels in a basket.

The above picture of unlabelled and mixed up colours of threads, shows how daunting it can be for someone who is colour blind to pick out a particular colour or shade of thread.

The limitations in sewing are that you may not know which colours go with which in this modern world. The answer is not, don't sew, but share the project and get help where you need it.

Some cross stich can be a little more difficult, as can dress making and creating home accessories. It is not necessarily the making of something, but usually the use of colour. For example, by starting small and adding things as you grow in confidence, there are many things you can do. It is probably not wise to work in a complicated range of browns or greens, if this is your colour bar, as it can be difficult to tell them apart.

If working on a garment, make sure that the tacking stitch stands out well from the garment and that you can see it clearly. The diagram below shows how a light thread stands out against a dark fabric.

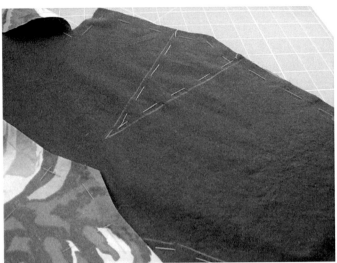

Picture showing a garment with tacking stitches to secure the fabric.

If using a thread to join things then it is a good idea to ask a trusted friend, who has full colour vision, to agree with your choice of matching colour thread. If you are making cushions or chair covers, it is best to discuss the colour choice of fabric as well as threads used, to achieve the desired impact. In this way full colour sighted people can appreciate your work too. All your friends can be impressed by your beautiful handiwork and how it compliments your room.

In a way it is like having half of a puzzle. As soon as you join with someone to help you, with the missing piece becoming the choice of colours, then the whole thing becomes clearer and easier.

- If your child is colour blind they can still sew.
- If using tacking stitches, make sure the colour thread stands out from the garment fabric easily.
- Help and advice on colour choices will be needed.
- Always try and give advice on colours that your son or daughter likes. That way they can enjoy the results of their labours as well as others appreciating the finished product.

Colour blindness and sport.

This is an interesting topic. Sport is about more than playing a game. It is about how we play and what rules we follow, but it is also important to realise how colour affects our performance.

If I play snooker or billiards or pool, then colour comes into the equation. With pool, the balls are fairly easy to tell apart if you have some colour vision as one set has a two tone colour system. When considering billiards where there are only three balls, then again so long as one uses colours that you can know apart it is not too hard.

However, when considering snooker, then it can be difficult but not impossible. The trick with snooker is to memorise where the ball or balls you don't know are at all times. I understand that this is exactly what Peter Ebdon and Mark Williams do when they play Snooker tournaments. They can also ask the referee if they have *'lost'* one of the balls.

The balls that normally cause the problem are the green and brown balls that can sometimes be confused with each other or the red balls. My father used to love snooker, he would always say that if he tried to pot a ball and it stayed up then it was a red, but if it went down then the chances were that it was a green or a brown!

Many years ago, I read a comic book with a team in it called *'Legges Eleven'*. They were a local football team of amateurs as I remember. When they started playing, they noticed that their goal keeper would not always know which players were on which team during certain matches. It transpired that the goal keeper was colour blind and couldn't always tell which colour shirt was on his team. In the end, they felt the best thing to do was to add a lightening type of strip on their tops so that whichever team they played, he could not confuse the colours of the tops.

This is an interesting thing as I know that some children find it difficult to recognise some colours. This is quite common not just with red, brown and green, but also with types of blues like purple. Indeed purple does look hard to distinguish as a colour for some people with that colour spectrum deficiency as it can be confused with black. Blues and aquas or limes can also be quite difficult.

The problem is that at a distance, some colours are harder to see for anyone who is colour blind. Even those picking out far away targets may well find it difficult to discern colours too. The problem is not that you can't see, but that you are not sure which colour is which. When you add poor light into the equation then an object can become a blur of colour, so that you cannot see anything but a general shade. I never know what colour buoys are in the sea. Even bird spotting can be challenging and I admit I am not really good at it. Seeing the colour of animals at a distance can be hard too. It is one thing to see something up close, but another to see it a long way away.

- Colour discernment in the sport arena can be challenging.
- You can still play snooker and other table sports but learn to watch the brown and green balls. Always ask if you are not certain.
- You can still play sport to a high standard and even turn professional.
- Make sure schools are aware if your child has difficulty with certain colours.
- Train your child in observation so that they are not just reliant on colour for discerning types of birds or plants too.

Chapter 7 - Frequently Asked Questions

Note: To help you find the specific information you need quickly, some information in the FAQ section will repeat some of the points already discussed. I have also occasionally referred back to some of the chapters in the book for more detailed information.

Can girls be colour blind?

This is a question I have often heard discussed. The answer to this is yes. Although more boys are colour blind than girls it is definitely possible as I can prove since I was born with this condition.

Colour blindness is not dependent on gender but on inherited genes. It happens when the cones or rods in the eye either don't function properly or they are absent.

To understand why, we need to go back to consider what colour is and how we see it. Colour is something that many take for granted. However in layman's terms, colour is an interpretation by our eyes of how we see light. This is like a rainbow, which changes colour as light filters through the sky after a downpour of rain. Basically, just as sound is interpreted by our brains from audio wavelengths we hear with our ears, so colour is interpreted by light wavelengths we see with our eyes. Just as some people cannot hear a full range of sounds, so some people cannot see a full range of colour.

This can happen to girls as well as boys but it is more common for boys to have colour blindness than girls. To understand this we must go back to basic biology and the study of genetics. Colour blindness is carried on the X chromosomes. As we know a boy has one X chromosome and one Y chromosome whereas girls have two X chromosomes.

For a boy to be colour blind he only needs the one X that carries colour blindness to be affected, but a girl needs to have both her X chromosomes to carry the colour blindness for her to be colour blind. This is because if a girl inherits only one chromosome that is affected, then she will use the fully functioning X chromosome to see colours in the same way as full colour sighted people. In this instance, the affected X chromosome will be what is known as *'recessive'* (in other words it will be dormant). For more information, see the write up and diagrams titled Genetic Inheritance in the chapter on Colour Blindness on Page 21.

Can adults become colour blind?

It is rare for adults to become colour blind later on in life, but not impossible. Colour blindness is usually something that is inherited through our genes but it can come as a result of an illness or an accident that affects our eyes. The daughter of a friend of mine once had her colour vision become mixed up. She saw the sky as green and the grass as blue. Fortunately this was a temporary thing which didn't make her colour blind but did upset how she viewed things for a while before her vision returned to normal. I believe this was the result of very bright lights.

Colours can also be temporarily lost during eye operations, especially when dealing with the retina. This normally clears up once the eye had fully repaired.

Some older people find their eyesight can change s they get older, but usually their brains remember the way colour used to look and so they aren't affected in quite the same way. Their need for more light though can change some of their colour perception.

What causes colour blindness?

Colour blindness is usually inherited in your genes. However it can also be the result of illness, or aging. It can also be as the result of a number of eye problems such as glaucoma and diabetic retinopathy. Even macular degeneration and cataracts can be instrumental in leading to colour blindness. Then again there is always the injury to the head caused by a bump, damage to an eye or even the side effects of medicines. Some of these causes only lead to temporary colour blindness, but others can be more long term.

This really highlights the need for good medical care when there are injuries, but also regular check-ups for eyesight and general health. Many people find that with age they need more light to see well. Older people may have their colour vision affected by age and light too. However, it is rare for them to become what is known as colour blind. This is because their brain remembers how they used to see colour. It therefore compensates for their lack of colour discernment and the reduction of light and how that affects their colour vision.

Is there a treatment for colour blindness?

If colour blindness has come during a lifetime then it may have a medical cause such as cataracts, or another eye problem caused by diabetes or an injury to the head or even by some medications. If this is the case then a doctor's assistance is needed or that of an optician.

If however, the colour blindness is an inherited case, there is not much that can be done to cure it, but there are things one can do to help the eyes. Many people with colour blindness are sensitive to light so using a good pair of sunglasses can be beneficial, or even a sunhat to help shade the eyes. Care with computer screens should be considered too, since reducing glare and eyestrain can be very helpful and there are again special glasses that can be used to help protect the eyes when using computer screens. Other options are learning to live with colour blindness and how best to help a person who is affected in this way.

Colour blindness is not life-threatening, but there are many things you can do to help. One of them is to promote understanding about the condition. Some countries believe that if you are colour blind, there are few jobs you can do. This is not necessarily true. As the section in this book on colour blindness at work on page 32 shows, there is no reason to not work or drive a vehicle, so long as you can use a coping mechanism. There is perhaps the exception of a pilot's licence (where you need to see different landing lights to land your airplane) or other similar jobs.

My dad and I always had a rhyme for traffic lights which many use

'At the top you stop (Red),
in the middle you get ready (Amber),
and below you go (Green)'.

I know that when Red and Amber light up together it indicates that you are getting ready to stop, but I have never found that a problem. The only time I have found traffic lights difficult was when they were in full sun, but then most people find this difficult. In those situations it is important to be aware of what is happening around you.

Below is a very interesting picture. It is a set of traffic lights from Canada. As you can see, the positions of shape are used to help colour blind people to know more quickly which light is which, a very interesting idea.

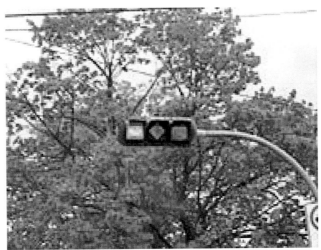

A set of traffic lights in Canada.

The key thing is to recognise that some people may have these sorts of challenges and we can allow for them. This is like having a ramp as well as stairs for those in a wheel chair, or writing the name of a colour on a garment, there is often a simple solution. The thing is that many people are slightly colour blind and don't even know!

Is there a cure for colour blindness?

To be honest, I don't think there can be one since it is not an illness. It is generally caused by an inherited gene, and we don't really understand enough about how it works to provide a correction for it. The important thing is to be correctly diagnosed. This is because it is not always caused by genetic inheritance but could be the result of an injury, medication, or even an eye condition like cataracts. One day, scientists may come up with a solution, but I don't think we are close to that point yet. After all, the way we see colour is quite complicated. I think they have done well just to understand how our eyes enable our brains to process so much information, let alone come up with a way to correct colour vision. This is especially because there are so many variations in the way we 'see' colour.

Is there a connection between cataracts and colour blindness?

Cataracts are known to distort our view of colours. The suggestion that cataracts are a form of colour blindness is a myth. I know of people who have experienced a change in their view of colours, but it is thought that the vibrancy of colours is reduced rather than lost. It would mean that some colours, if not colours in general, would seem a little duller. Due to the reduced light entering the eye, everything the eye 'sees' would be affected and this would change the brain's interpretation of things viewed too. In fact I have heard people who have had cataracts say that cobwebs seem to miraculously appear when full vision is restored. The impact of cataracts is usually quite slow as they develop over a period of time. However, most full colour vision is generally restored on the removal of the cataracts. This would indicate that colour vision is impaired rather than lost or not functioning. For more information, see the chapter on 'Colour Blindness' on Page 11.

What are the symptoms of colour blindness?

When children are small, colour blindness can be hard to spot. There will be tell-tale signs, but it will take a while for you to be certain. As you start to interact with a child, then their colour preferences become more noticeable. Be aware of what colours they favour. When they are small, they may respond to certain coloured toys more than others. As they grow it will become more obvious. They will be slow to know some colours and may confuse others. They may not be sure which toy brick is brown or green and may mix them up. Sometimes pink may be seen as a type of blue.

It is important to be patient when teaching children colours and always to be aware that their lack of response or confusion may be because of colour blindness. Remember, if they are colour blind then they are unable to learn the colours because they cannot see them as you do.

As soon as they are old enough, there are pictures on the internet that you can use to help you discover whether or not they are actually colour blind. These tests are called *'Ishihara'* tests. There is more information on these tests on my website, **www.colourblindnesstips.com**. There are also photographs that show how you see a picture and how someone sees it with a different colour view. These are also on my website. They are actually film clips and I think they are brilliant. When I saw them I was amazed!

For the first time, my husband could see some of the world as I saw it. No need to describe a colour. He finally could have a real idea of what I could see. I really recommend looking at these clips. With children you can always ask them if they can see any difference between them. If they have that colour bar, then they will not see the difference between the pictures.

As children grow up, you will see that they like some colours more than others. This will impact their clothes choices or their preferences for coloured pictures. For my husband and me it was quite easy. I knew what they would see if they were colour blind (being colour blind myself).

I already knew that our daughter would not be colour blind but would carry the affected gene, while our son was bound to be colour blind. This was because my husband was not colour blind and so would pass a clear X chromosome to our daughter, while I would pass an affected X chromosome as I am colour blind (which means both my X chromosomes carry colour blindness). Our son naturally inherited the Y chromosome from his father but the affected X chromosome from me. For more information on inherited colour blindness see the chapter on Genetic Inheritance on Page 21.

Adults often develop techniques for hiding their colour blindness and this makes it harder to realise that they are colour blind. People often hide it because of the lack of understanding of others. Sometimes people do not know they are colour blind. In days gone by, we said that someone was *'not good with colours'*. Nowadays I think it is better to be aware that there are people who are colour blind and we should make allowances for it, rather than ridicule or deny it.

Are there special glasses for colour blindness?

There some glasses called Oxy-Iso glasses. These glasses are designed to help people with red-green colour blindness. When I looked at a review on these glasses, the comparison view it showed me (a picture showing a scene with and without using the glasses) seemed to make the colours a little deeper and reduce the glare. The change was quite strange and I don't think I could wear them for long periods. The thing is, you get used to seeing what you can see. It's not like corrective viewing for long or short sightedness. For me it is still in the *'maybe one day'* list of things rather than in the *'must get now'* range. However, they are available to buy on the internet, so feel free to look them up for yourself and see what you feel about their possible uses.

What is Colour blindness?

Colour blindness is an inability to 'see' certain colour ranges. It is usually the result of an inherited condition, an illness or damage to the head that affects the way the brain interprets what the eyes see. Colour is actually 'perceived' by the brain as light waves that the eye sees through its cones and rods. This is then interpreted as a colour depending on the light waves seen.

Basically, we see at least three colour wave bands with the cones in our eyes: - Red, Blue and Green. Then there is another part of our eye known as rods which see temperatures. This is all interpreted by the eye as colours. If any of our cones or rods are malfunctioning, or even not present, then we cannot 'see' all colours in the same way as everyone else.

We cannot learn to see colours as we do not have the ability to interpret them. This is because the receptors in our eyes that pick up the light waves are not all functioning, or some may be missing. This does not mean that we are blind but that certain colours are hard to distinguish from others. This may be because we cannot see the same depth of colour as others, but we can see colour, just not quite in the same way as others. However, there are another group of people who can only see varying shades of grey. This is much rarer but can be inherited, as well as the result of illness or accident. This group of people will only see in black and white or varying shades of grey. For further information see the chapter on Colour Blindness on Page 11.

What is the 'Unwritten Code'?

The 'Unwritten Code' refers to all the messages that are written in colour. Nature has them in abundance. We have tended to adopt these colours in everyday use from signs to the colour of objects which those with full colour vision instinctively know.

Consider the colour green. This is used as a colour for go on traffic lights and also for enter on card machines. People who can see the colour green can find the start or go button quicker than colour blind people. We will find the button but it is harder for us to be certain that we are pressing the right one. I would be useless at touch typing by colour!

Red is used as a warning colour and so everyone knows that red means danger but not all of us can be sure of the colour. We look at the object like a fire engine. Then there is yellow and black. The bee and the wasp have these colours and we use them as warning colours in Airports to point the way or warn of slippery areas. Have you noticed that most direction or information type signs on the road are in blue and danger ones like stop signs are in red? Entry and exits of motorways are defined by green and red lights.

When shopping, those with full colour sight can find their sizes easily by scanning the colour of labels on clothes while those with colour blindness have to read the labels. Then there are products set up in shops according to colour. Like the tops of milk or the labels on other food products declaring the percentages of fat. Even butter and spreads seem to have their own language of colour.

It is in this way that those of us who are colour blind are a little slower to see things as we cannot use colour to guide us. We have to follow other clues and learn to interpret the colour messages in other ways. I suppose it is like playing a computer game. We cannot read the colour clues that tell us what to do next as quickly as others. We may not know that all the people in that group are a shade of green and that I have to shoot them. I have to wait for them to shoot me to know I need to defend myself.

Naomi Davies

How is colour blindness inherited?

This is an important question as understanding how it is inherited can help in the understanding of colour blindness itself. Colour blindness is not usually something that just happens (unless the result of an illness, or accident, that affects the eyes or the part of the brain that interprets our colour vision), but it is something that is inherited. This means that it is not something we can eradicate by learning or the use of eye aids like glasses or contact lenses (at present glasses and contact lenses do not give full normal colour vision). If you cannot see something, then you cannot see it.

Colour blindness is carried on the X chromosome. A boy inherits one X chromosome from his mother and a Y chromosome from his father. A girl inherits two X chromosomes, one from her father and one from her mother. For a boy to be colour blind, he needs to inherit an affected X chromosome from his mother. For a girl to be colour blind, she needs both her X chromosomes to be affected. This is because the X chromosome is recessive and the non-affected X chromosome will over-ride the affected one.

So if a colour seeing man marries a colour seeing woman, then neither of their children should be colour blind. However, if the woman has a recessive X chromosome that carries the colour blindness then it could be different. If the son inherits the affected X chromosome then he will be colour blind. If the daughter inherits it then she will carry the colour blindness but not be colour blind herself. In this way it can be a surprise if a son is colour blind when neither of the parents have this condition. About 7% of boys are born colour blind.

With regard to a girl being colour blind, this is rarer and affects only about 0.4%. This can only happen if the father is colour blind and the mother passes an affected X chromosome to the daughter. If mum passes a clear X chromosome, then the daughter will carry it from her father but not be colour blind herself.

It can be very confusing but suffice to say, it is much rarer for girls than boys to be born colour blind, but not impossible. For further information, see the Chapter on Genetic Inheritance on Page 21.

Are there contact lenses for colour blindness?

This is something that is being considered but as there are a number of types of colour blindness, it can be quite difficult to find a good solution. Indeed, some reports say it can distort your vision and may not be considered safe for regular use. From what I can gather, the vision given by these contact lenses is not the same as for sight correction and cannot give full colour restoration. Our colour vision is very specialised. We all have so many different variations of colour vision which are dependent on how our brains interpret the light waves that we see. Looking at these variations of what we can see, it soon becomes evident that there is no quick and easy fix.

This is obviously a work in progress and it may well be that a solution will become available. In the meantime, I personally feel we would be wise to discover our own methods of colour discernment. This will help us to see things in the world to the best of our abilities. With care and an awareness of our own individual view of colour, we can find our own various coping mechanisms. These will enable us to live as normal a life as possible in our colour co-ordinated world.

Do you know any famous people who are colour blind?

There are indeed many people who are famous and are colour blind. It is just something that is not often talked about. Just as some athletes are known to have coped with diabetes, such as Sir Steve Redgrave the Olympian Rower. Who would have believed that Mark Spitz the Olympic Swimmer who also won a number of medals could have coped with asthma? Both these men performed remarkable achievements which were noteworthy even without their own health challenges. To achieve these goals while dealing with medical issues, only serves to make them more remarkable. Mark won a lot of medals in one year, while Sir Steve won medals in five successive Olympic Games. To succeed in these ways with their health challenges is just amazing. These examples prove that what sets you apart from others is how you cope or deal with your own issues and life challenges.

As an encouragement, here are a few people that I have been reliably informed are colour blind and have not let it stop them achieving things. These are people that I have found out about through my own research of information that is readily available to the general public. There will be more, but as I said, it is not something that is generally talked about. I would hope that in time, more people would share the reality of their colour blindness. In this way, more and more of us would realise that colour blindness does not need to stop us achieving our goals, or having an impact on our peers.

- **John Dalton** – a chemist from the 1700s who discovered and did a lot of work on colour blindness. He is responsible for much of our understanding on the topic. He was also involved in early work on the understanding of the atom.

- **Anthony Burgess** – a British author. The pen name of John Anthony Burgess Wilson who wrote historical fiction and was a playwright, screen writer, travel writer, broadcaster, and linguist. He was awarded the *'Commandeur des Arts et des Lettres'* of France, as well as being a Fellow of the Royal Society of Literature.

- **Bill Clinton** – The 42nd President of the United States of America. At 46 years old, he was the third youngest president of the USA and he has had an enormous influence on the world as we know it.

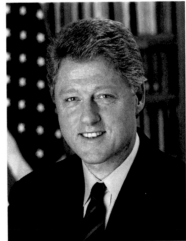

Bill Clinton

- **Bob Dole** – Former senator in America also active in American politics.

- **Tom Watts** – an American musician. He plays an assortment of instruments and publishes music on his own label.

- **George Michael** – a British Musician. He started with *'Wham'* and is remembered for a number of songs singing with Elton John and also Aretha Franklin.

- **William Hague** – a British Politician and Member of Parliament who has held a number of posts in government, including as leader of the Conservative Party.

- **Paul Newman** – an American actor who was well known and very successful in his career. Remembered for *'The Sting'* and *'Butch Cassidy and the Sundance Kid'*, just to name a couple.

- **Rutger Hauer** – a famous actor. When he left the Dutch Navy, he went on to follow in his parents footsteps as an actor of renown and acted in films like *'Scorcher'*, *'Blade Runner'*, *'Never Enough'*, *'Batman Begins'*. He also went on to be a Director and Producer and adapt *'Of Mice and Men'* by John Steinbeck for the stage.

- **Meat Loaf** – a very successful musician and entertainer. Born in the USA he has sung and acted to great acclaim. Songs like *'I'd Do Anything for Love (But I Won't Do That)'* and acting in *'The Rocky Horror Show'* to mention one of his best known parts.

- **Bing Crosby** – one of the most successful and well known singers, actors, and entertainers. Always remembered for the song *'White Christmas'* and acting with his friend the great comedian Bob Hope.

- **Keanu Reeves** – another successful musician and all round actor. He plays the guitar and acted in films like *'Speed'*, *'Bill and Ted'*, *'The Matrix'* (to name just a few).

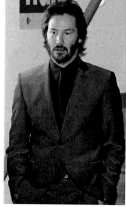

Keanu Reeves

- **Fred Rogers** – real name Fred McFeely Rogers. A renowned educator, songwriter, author, television host and Presbyterian minister.

- **Jack Nicklaus** – a well-known and respected successful golfer. He was the winner of the Green Jacket in the *'US Masters'* golf tournament.

- **Matt Lauer** – named as best dressed man on a number of lists including Vanity Fair.

- **Mark Twain** – a renowned author who wrote some of the best known books like *'Hucklebury Finn'*.

- **Mark Williams** – Famous Snooker player (he memorises where balls are but anyone can ask if you *'lose'* the green or brown)

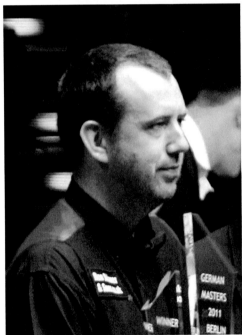
Mark Williams

- **Peter Ebdon** – Famous Snooker player (he will also note where the snooker balls are on the table – it is usually the brown or the green that cause the problems)

None of the above people were prevented from making an impact on the world because of their colour blindness. They may not have been able to do everything they wanted to do (Rutger Hauer could not progress as a sailor and so changed his career), or even had to change the way they served their country (Paul Newman wanted to be a pilot for the Navy but failed the colour test so he trained to be a radioman and a gunner before going on to be a successful actor). Bill Clinton and Bob Dole, both found it hard to know when they were appearing on camera during debates and so they used some special lights to tell them instead of the usual cues.

Is there a way to fix colour blindness?

This is a question that has puzzled scientists and those who experience colour blindness for a long time. Our understanding of colour and how we perceive it has led to amazing discoveries and inventions such as film, television, coloured woven thread, cross-stitch threads, paints, transmitted colour like on the internet, laser lights, and fireworks. Indeed there are many things we take for granted in our modern world that we have as a result of the research into colour blindness.

However, understanding how we see colour is one thing, but understanding how to *'fix'* colour vision is another. It isn't the same thing as corrective glasses for long or short sightedness. Neither is it comparable with hearing aids that replace the sounds we can't hear. Although even with hearing aids there are still problems. They are a great help but there is still room for improvement as sometimes all sound is increased and not just the missing or reduced ones.

The difficulty with colour vision, is that there are many ways in which it can be impaired. They range from illness and drugs to damage to the head. Then there is the inherited form. There are so many things that can change the way we see colour, that there cannot easily be one fix. We need to understand so much more about how the different permutations of colour vision work, before we can find a way of correcting them.

There are lots of ideas from contact lenses to glasses but we have not come up with a total solution yet. Many people like me, have found ways of coping. We have learnt to accept that while we may not see the same as others, what we do see is also beautiful.

Who discovered colour blindness?

At first glance, this is not an easy question to answer. Obviously the first person to discover colour blindness was the first person to realise that people saw things differently. However, many of us see things differently to other people. It may be because of the way we were brought up but also the way we understand the world.

The name of the man who is accredited with doing the first real work on colour blindness is John Dalton. He was born in the September of 1766 and died in 1844, before even my parents were born. He was a scientist and published his paper on *'Extraordinary facts relating to the vision of colours'* in 1793.

He started working as a teacher but became interested in meteorology and mathematics. Both he and his brother were colour blind in the red-green spectrum. He was naturally intrigued by the way he and his brother saw colours compared to other people.

He thought it was due to the liquid in the eyeball and donated his eyes for research after his death. He wanted another scientist to check his theory that the liquid was coloured and so impacted the way we see colours. The follow up experiments on his eyes disproved this part of his theory. Later, it was revealed that the problem was in the perception of colour, rather than the eye itself.

However, his notes on the seeing of colour were obviously helpful as he is thought of as the first person to do any real scientific research on colour sight, and many refer to colour blindness as Daltonism.

During his life he was a respected chemist and one of the early contributors in the field of atomic theory. So being colour blind does not mean being stupid, or that you cannot make a valuable contribution to whatever line of work you do, or life you lead.

Are there different types of colour blindness?

There are a number of what are known as colour bars. There is the Red, the Blue and the Green. There is also monochrome vision (where one sees only Greys). The thing to remember with colour vision, is that because we see colour when our brain interprets the light waves, it is very hard to put things in easy packages like colour bars.

Those who have some colour vision (who are officially colour blind) will see different versions of colour. I think my dad had it right when he said that we didn't see the depth of colours, although this is a simplified version of what we actually see. If you look at my website, **www.colourblindnesstips.com** you will see films showing how differently we see things with different colour bars.

I personally think that we need to look at how we create colours. Firstly we have Primary, Secondary and Tertiary types of colour.

Primary Colours.

These are Red, Blue and Yellow along with Black (an absence of colour) and White (a multiplicity of colour). These are the basic building blocks of colour.

Secondary Colours

This is where two of the primary colours are used to create a new colour. For example we use red and yellow to make orange or blue and yellow to make green.

Tertiary Colours

This next group consists of colours that are made when mixing three primary colours. An example of this is brown which is created when mixing Red, Yellow and Blue.

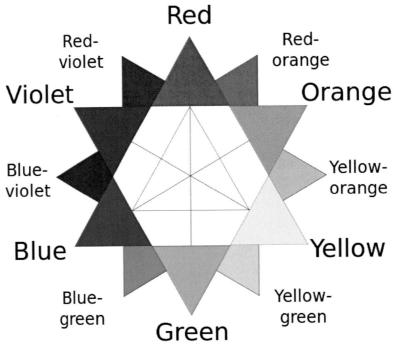

A traditional RYB colour wheel.

The above palette of colour is the same one as I used at school showing red, yellow and blue. In art class we added white and black. We used the paints in powder form and added water.

As you can see, by mixing red and yellow, we get orange. By mixing yellow and blue, we get green. Thus you can see we mix a lot of basic colours to get many of what we think of as simple, everyday colours.

From this brief look at how we create colours with paint, it becomes obvious that it is quite difficult for a person who is colour blind to be certain of any colour. Since green (one of the main colour bars) is made from mixing primary colours yellow and blue, and red (another common colour bar) is used in the mixing of other colours like orange, it becomes evident that someone who is colour blind will have a problem discerning some of the colours. The impaired cones or rods will not send sufficiently accurate messages to the brain, which in turn will not always make a correct judgement call on the information presented. In other words, if you are colour blind you cannot really be certain of any colour since the information is incomplete.

However, this does not mean that a person who is colour blind cannot create their own interpretation of how they see colours. This ability is quite useful, e.g. when baking something like biscuits I look for my own interpretation of 'fawn' so that I know they are baked.

When cooking other things, I use timing to help me know when things are cooked as well as my sense of smell and taste. I have never allowed my colour bar to hold me back and have just found inventive ways around it as mentioned earlier in this book under the chapter on 'Living with Colour Blindness' on Page28 . I have just learned to tune into other indicators so that I know what is going on around me. I have always disliked the phrase 'can't' for me it is 'how else can I sort this?'.

Are women better with colours than men?

It has been suggested that about 2 or 3 % of women may have a fourth cone and so have what is known as 'tetrachromatic' vision. This gives them a much better sense of colour differences and means that they are better at arranging and matching colours. If you consider that about 7% of men are colour blind and 0.4% of women, then it will probably follow that on balance women are better than men at dealing with colours.

However, there will always be exceptions as this cannot be an exact science. We are still learning about colour and how best to see it, yet alone how best to use our knowledge of colour. Indeed, there are probably many other factors that influence the reality that many women are excellent homemakers. In general it is women who look after the decorating and furnishing of their homes. Even so, there are also many men who are very good at this as well and some of them may have this extra cone too; I am just looking at the overall picture.

How or when can you test for colour blindness? As a toddler or child or adult

It is fairly easy to test for colour blindness once we are older. There are patterns with hidden numbers and drawings known as *'Ishihara'* tests.

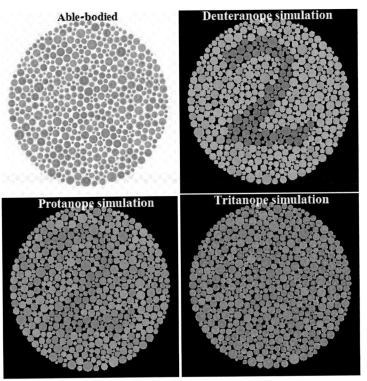

Examples of Ishihara tests.

With regard to the above pictures, the only number I can see clearly is the '2' in the top right hand corner picture. I am aware that there is something in the others, but I cannot make it out as clearly. I could however make a reasonable guess at the answer and can trace roughly where it is. The top left picture however, simply looks like a coloured pattern of dots. In a way, the fact that I can almost see the number in the two lower diagrams gives strength to my point on Pages 52-53, that because our colours are made up from others, it is hard to be certain of any colour. My colour vision is obviously affected by more than one colour bar since all colours impact on our view or 'seeing' of colour – as illustrated by the RYB colour wheel on Page 52.

If you are colour blind then you see one thing but if you have full colour vision then you will see different things. You can find out more about these tests on my website **www.colourblindnesstips.com**

However, with very young children testing is a little more difficult. The best way is to look for colour preferences and to see how they respond to colour choices as they learn their colours. Although many girls preferred pink I preferred blue. It is also interesting to see what colours they respond to and what pictures they think appealing. These are all indicators but certainty can only come as they grow and start to learn colours and are able to do the *'Ishihara'* test.

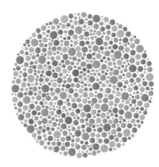

Looking at this picture above, I cannot see anything other than a random display of coloured dots! My husband assures me that in this diagram, and the one above, there is something to be seen!

Does colour affect our eating or buying habits or other choices?

This is something that all marketers know the answer to and it is a definite yes. We are influenced by colours in packaging and the presentation of food and many other things.

Blue is a known appetite suppressant. Red is known as a prohibitive colour and is often used to warn of danger as with traffic lights or red warning signs on roads or beaches. Green is a more permissive colour and encourages us to relax. Indeed green is one of the most often used colours in nature, and known to be a restful colour to the eyes. Some colours make us feel happy while others make us feel bold.

We all have colours that we regard as our own favourites. We like to wear different colours that we feel suit us more than others. Then there is the colour combination of yellow and black that creates a feeling of fear. This is possibly why we react so much to bees and wasps, as the fear of being stung or hurt is very much more real to some than others.

Colour is also evident in cultural choices. In western countries red and green are symbols of Christmas. Green was a sacred colour to Egyptians as they looked forward to spring. I am also told that green is sacred to Muslims and that the Japanese Emperor Hirohito's birthday was called *'Green Day'* as he loved to garden.

In China, brides do not generally choose white as it is their colour for mourning while in western countries black is considered a mourning colour.

So you can see that there are cultural differences to the way we use and respond to colours too. Colour is a very emotive subject.

What is the importance of colour?

The shade of a colour is important. The deeper and more prime a colour is the more chance even those who are colour blind can cope or discern it. The world we live in is full of colour. Many companies use it extensively in their brochures and displays. A colour blind person may not appreciate all the effects of colour as they do not generally see the depth of colours displayed.

It is important to be aware of colours as they are used to give out messages. It is important for those who are colour blind to know about this and to develop their own way of interpreting the messages.

With traffic lights, they need to know that:

'at the top you stop,
in the middle you get ready,
and below you go'.

The fact that they may not know what each colour is called is not as important as knowing what the lights are telling them.

It can be pointed out at an early age that road signs with a blue back ground are mostly for information, whereas red signs usually denote some kind of danger. This sort of early help will enable them to be more aware and look at signs in a more informed way. At airports, it is helpful to know that certain colours on signs can have different meanings e.g. yellow and black can be warnings (some slippery signs are in these colours).

Our son had a lot of early help through his nursery school providing the colour table. Each week there was a different colour and everyone brought in an object of that colour. It will have taught him that a colour can have lots of shades and still be the same colour. It will also have helped him to recognise and be aware of more colour messages than he might otherwise have been. This is not to say that he could be treated or cured of colour blindness, rather that he was able to develop more of his own ideas of how he viewed colour and has been able to use this information throughout his life.

How can we help people in their everyday life who are colour blind?

The way we use colour means that we need to allow for people who are colour blind. Just as we introduce slopes and lifts for people who struggle with stairs, so we need to introduce alternatives for people who cannot perceive all colours. Colour is everywhere but how we use it is important.

At work with a colour coded diary, it is easy to introduce shapes with colours so that all triangles might be red and all circles might be yellow. This way both a colour sighted person and a colour blind person can respond to the diary information with ease.

Where it is not so easy to introduce an extra guide, it is important to make sure that signs such as those in airports are large with clear markings like black writing on yellow so that everyone can follow them. When setting up appliances with colour coded buttons and colour instructions, it is important to allow for people to work out which is which, even if they can't be sure which colour is red or green. For example, it is quite easy to print the word *'enter'* rather than say press the *'green'* button on machines like card readers.

The shade of a colour is also important. The deeper and more prime a colour is, the more chance there is that even those who are colour blind can cope. With traffic lights then one can learn the positions of the colours and know the sequence, so there are many innovative ways of knowing which one to follow, although some people will need a little longer than others.

With computers, it is important to remember that there are three ranges of colour - primary, secondary and tertiary. It is when one mixes the palette that colours are harder to decipher. The arrangement or diagram on a computer may look very pretty but may not always be very serviceable for someone who is colour blind.

It must be remembered that not everyone knows they are colour blind and may not discover it until later in life. Children in particular should be protected from misinformation relating to colour. I was once in a school as a student teacher, when members of staff discovered that one of their boys was colour blind. Unfortunately they had used colour very heavily in their maths program so that it had impeded his learning of mathematics!

What many of them in the school obviously didn't then know, is that around 7% of the boys and 0.4% of their girls were likely to have been affected too. I admit this was back in the sixties and hopefully people are more aware of the impact of colour now than they were in those days.

What does a colour blind person see?

To say that a colour blind person doesn't see the depth of colour is not always helpful. The problem is that it is hard to describe colour, without using the reference of colour. How do you describe the redness of red without likening it to another colour, or saying one red is more crimson and another more scarlet?

The picture below shows some fruit. The apples on the left are coloured red on the top and green on the bottom. The two apples on the right are two distinct shades of green. This is what my husband can see when he looks at the pictures. To me however, the left apples look red and the apples on the right look green. This is just an everyday example of how our colour vision can impact our lives. I always have to be careful when buying fresh fruit and vegetables and often shop with my husband or with a friend I know well.

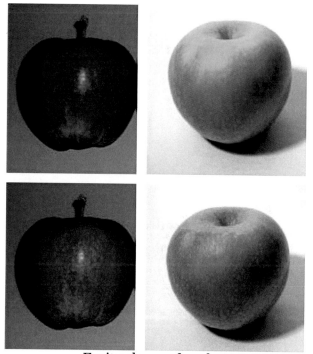

Fruit colours of apples.

I have recently discovered some comparison films showing what someone with a red bar can see compared to full colour vision. Similarly there are ones for other colour spectrums. You can find some on my website **www.colourblindnesstips.com**

I found this fascinating when I sat down and viewed these film clips with my husband. For the first time, he could see the differences between his colour vision and mine. Truly amazing! One obvious regret is that I could not sit down with my late father and mother, so that we could share this latest insight into how we see colour!

What a colour blind person can see is dependent on the type of colour blindness they have inherited. Some people can only see in mono chrome which is actually shades of grey. I can see more than this, so I can only imagine that for them it is like watching the old black and white televisions, which showed various shades of grey.

There are also some who have problems with certain colours like Red Brown & Green. Some have problems with Blues & Yellows. To understand more we need to go back to art class and consider the make-up of colours.

I was taught that there are five primary colours. These are; Black, White, Red, Blue & Yellow. Now Black is regarded as an absence of colour, while White is thought of as a mixture of all colours. It is the Red Blue & Yellow that are more interesting.

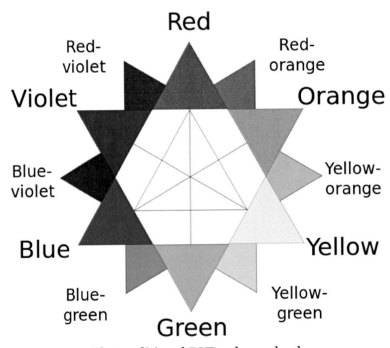

The traditional RYB colour wheel.

I was taught that if I wanted to make the colour pink, I would take the red and add white until I achieved the shade I wanted. If I wanted to make the colour green then I would mix blue & yellow. Again, if I wanted to make the colour orange then I would mix red & yellow, and so on.

I am sure by now, you are starting to realize that the mixture of these colours could make it difficult to identify which colour is which, if you cannot see or recognize any of the primary colours. This is why so many people find it difficult to match aqua type colours and lilacs. It doesn't however mean that they are necessarily colour blind. The problem is that as colour depends on light waves, our perception of them will vary depending on the light where we are viewing them. That's why it is so difficult to carry a particular colour in our heads, even when we have good colour vision. Now just as some people have amazingly superb hearing, so some people have amazing colour perception.

My father once explained to me that he didn't think we saw the depth of colour like others. This is another way of explaining it, that it is how we see the light waves. My children had a colour toy made up of plastic rings of different colours stacked on a pole. Sometimes I could see the one ring as green but at other times the light made it difficult to tell from brown or red. I knew the colour was different but I wasn't sure which was which, until I stacked them and could remember the colour order, but I was never really sure.

I always had to be very careful when mentioning colour to my son when he was little. As I was colour blind, I knew that I could give my son the wrong colour information. Fortunately, our daughter had normal colour vision and she and my husband could help me. At other times, I would memorise some of the toys that we had at home and their colours.

One of the regular questions I am asked when someone first knows I am colour blind is, *'What colour is this?'* If the object in question was one of the old letter or pillar boxes, then the answer was red. If it was grass then the answer was green, unless it was looking a little burnt or dark and then it might be brown. The problem is we cannot really describe a colour without using a colour. What colour is red unless it is crimson or scarlet or maybe a dark red or a light red?

What is a cone?

A cone is one of two types of 'photoreceptor cells' that are found in the retina of the eye. They help with our colour vision or perception of colour. Cones work best in bright light and perceive fine detail as well as rapid changes in images. There are a lot of these cones in the eye. The latest figures according to Wikipedia quoting *'Curcio et al'* from 1990 is an average of 4.5 million cones in the retina of the eye, basically there are a lot of them!

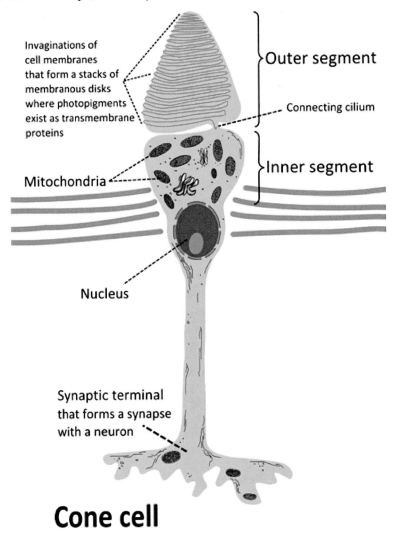

Invaginations of cell membranes that form a stacks of membranous disks where photopigments exist as transmembrane proteins

Outer segment

Connecting cilium

Inner segment

Mitochondria

Nucleus

Synaptic terminal that forms a synapse with a neuron

Cone cell

There are three types of cones. They operate to allow us to *'see'* three types of pigments. One absorbs blue (known as S cones as they pick up colours seen on the short wave of light transmission), while another type picks up green (known as M cones as these are on the medium band of light waves) and the third type collects red (known as L cones as these are on the long wave frequency). The fact that we have three types of cones in our eyes means that we have what is known as *'trichromatic'* vision. There have been reports of some people having *'tetrachromatic'* vision as these rare people have four or more types of cones. If any of the cones are affected by disease then this is serious, as destruction of the cones would lead to blindness.

What is a rod?

A rod is the second type of *'photoreceptor'* cells that are also found in the retina of the eye and are distinct from the cones. There are, according to Wikipedia who again quotes Oyster's textbook (1993) based on *'Curcio et al'* (1990), about 90 million of these rod cells packed into the retina of our eyes although some say there are approximately 125 million, so it is safe to say that there are a lot of them but probably more than cones!

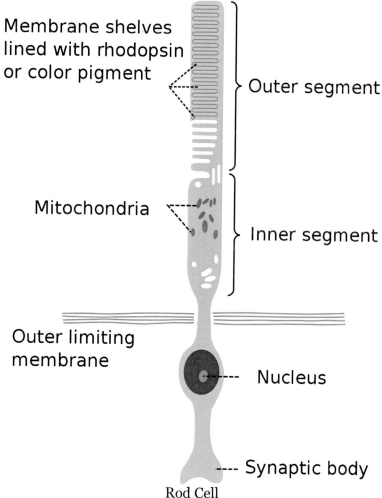

Rod Cell

The rods are very different to the cones and work best in dim light. As rods work best in dim light they are most active in night vision. They are also sensitive to temperature and may well help us to see warm and cold colours.

Where are cones & rods found?

The cones and rods are found in the retina of the eye. There are lots and lots of them packed into the retina together.

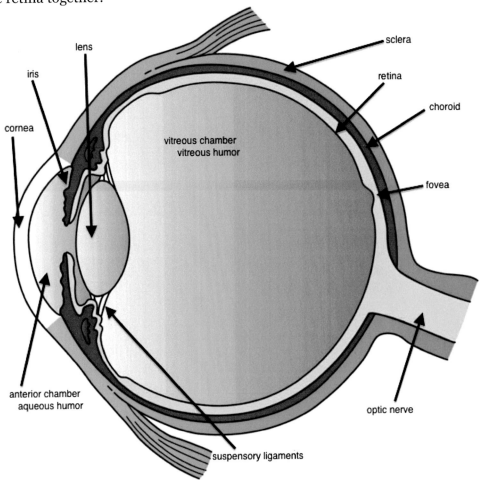

Above is a diagram of an eye showing the retina containing rods and cones

The retina is a thin coating that is around the interior of the eye. It is on the retina at the back of the eye, that the lens of the eye causes images to be reflected for the eye to 'see' them. The brain interprets these images aided by the cones and rods that are situated in the retina. Cones are fat and short, while rods are lean and long. The rods and cones help the brain to determine what the eye is seeing. The brain is like a computer that receives information in the form of light waves and it is the interpretation of these light waves that enable us to 'see' colour.

Do people dream in colour?

People's dreams are based on their everyday experiences. This means that everyone who knows what colour is, can dream in colour. It is how our brains interpret our dreams that enable us to see or remember what we dream. For someone who is colour blind, they can only dream with the colours as they 'see' them in their everyday lives.

Does the colour of our eyes affect colour blindness?

This is an interesting question that I was asked recently. The colour of our eyes is genetically inherited and is revealed to the world by the part of the eye known as the iris. Although in new born babies, the colour of the eye can change through a variety colours before settling on its final colour it is not connected to colour vision. Those people with 'albino eyes' have a condition known as 'photophobia' and have to be careful of over exposure to light. The iris in their eyes is sometimes pink rather than white and seems unable to filter light so that they need to protect their eyes.

However, the colour of the eyes is not what really affects colour vision. It is the receptors known as cones and rods in the eye that govern our colour vision. The three types of cone cell are responsible for the short wave lengths (known as the blue cone), the medium wave lengths (known as the green cone) and the long wave lengths (known as the red cone). The rod cell is responsible for our perception of temperature and intensity of colour.

If any these receptors are missing, malfunctioning or damaged then they cannot give us a full range of colour vision. Any disruption in this area can have an impact on our colour vision resulting in some form of colour blindness. More information can be found under the question *'What is colour blindness?'* on Page 46 and the chapter on *'Colour Blindness'* on Page 11.

Chapter 8 – Conclusion

I am a very positive person and I am always looking for a silver lining to any aspect of my life. For me, colour blindness is not a handicap of any kind, but a challenge. I know that I can never see colours as those with 'normal' colour vision, but I have no intention of allowing my colour blindness to limit me in any way. The achievements of those people like Sir Steve Redgrave who achieved so much in rowing regardless of the fact that he is a diabetic, inspire me. The chapter on 'Famous People' on Page 48 which lists worldwide contributors like John Dalton, Bill Clinton, Bing Crosby and others, merely confirms to me that it is our attitude and refusal to let colour blindness define us that is important. I hope I have been able to convey this positive outlook to you as a parent, as an interested friend, or as someone who is colour blind.

Even so, we still have much to learn about colour and how it impacts our lives. I think it is really important that we understand as much about colour and colour blindness as we can, so that we can dispel the myths and misunderstandings that exist about this topic.

I have written this book to help others who are colour blind. My aim was to show ways in which parents, teachers and others can help those of us who are colour blind. With care and a little ingenuity, we can live fulfilled lives. The lack of colour vision should not prevent us achieving our goals in an all colour seeing society. As the short section on 'famous people' shows, we can make a positive contribution and impact our world for good.

The research to understand how we see colour has had many benefits like colour television, computers and films in colour. It may yet one day lead to the ability to correct colour vision.

In the meantime, I hope that everyone who reads this book will realize that I have only touched on what I think are the most salient points. We are surrounded by colour in our modern world. There are so many everyday colour messages like *'press the green button'*, *'follow the red holiday signs'*, *'follow the green arrows'* on nature walks, etc. There are obviously far more areas than I have mentioned.

It is really important to think about how we use colour and how we need to allow for people who may not see the colour messages as quickly as others. I am hoping that any parent, teacher, employer, leader, friend, etc., will consider how to interpret the *'unwritten code'* of colour so that we can all enjoy and appreciate as much as possible from the gift of colour that we have and use every day of our lives.

Naomi Davies
www.colourblindnesstips.com

Appendix – Colour vision and animals

How do we test animals for colour vision?

This is done by behavioural tests. Although scientists can examine the colour receptors in the eyes of animals and insects to see what colours they are likely to see, a lot of testing is done by behavioural methods. For example, some soya milk or other delectable treat is put behind a particular coloured door or receptacle. The animal is rewarded by that particular treat when it uses or opens that particular door.

Do animals see the same as humans?

Different animals see different things dependant on their need. For example, eagles can see further than even humans. This is because of their need for distance view in the aid to finding their way at great speed and to enable them to hunt their prey. Hippos can see well under water. Geckos have brilliant night vision with colour. The fly has very special vision so that its eye sees all around. It sees things far quicker than humans, which explains why we find them so hard to swat. Scientists are still finding out about what animals 'see' and I am sure there is much more to discover about their vision. Since animals cannot speak to us and explain what they see, we have to observe and evaluate what they can see by the way they behave and respond to different situations.

Can animals be colour blind?

Animals see different things to humans. Domesticated animals such as cats and dogs are similar to rats and rabbits in that they have poor colour vision compared to humans. It would appear that they see mostly grey and perhaps some blue and yellow. Bulls are actually believed to be colour blind and re-act to the movement of the cape rather than the fact that it is red.

Other animals use colour to help them find food and hunt their prey as well as see those who would hunt them. For example those needing to know which fruits are ripe would need to distinguish between unripe and ripe berries.

Then there are those needing to see which plants will feed them and that they can pollinate. These are usually bees and butterflies. They seem to have the ability to see things we can't in the form of ultraviolet vision of the leaves, etc.

Then again there are hippos that can see under water, as well as alligators and crocodiles. There is even a diving bird which can see under water without the aid of goggles!

Some vipers respond to movement and sound while a pit viper is known to 'see' by feeling the temperature of an object or other creature.

Resources

Most of my resources have been from my own experience and speaking to many people during my life time. I have also used information that was generally available in my school biology classes. My intention was not to produce a scientific book but a practical understanding of how colour blindness exists and how best to help those affected by it.

My Website – **www.colourblindnesstips.com**

Wikipedia.org

Ishihara Colour Blindness Test

Fiction by Naomi Davies

As well as writing this book on Colour Blindness, Naomi has published four romantic novellas in the Sixty Minute Romance Series.

Love's Dilemma – Naomi Davies

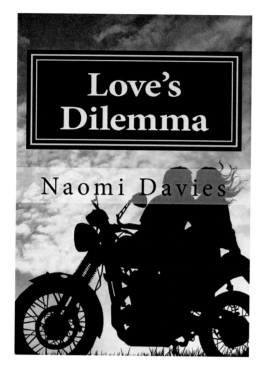

The fourth novella in the Sixty Minute Romance series

Plot Introduction...

Clair's whole life has been governed and controlled by a strict religious upbringing. She lives by a set of rules that she had no part in making. Clair also has a prodigious talent. She can sing like an angel. Her singing leads her to meet Max who is wild and free. He is alive and out of control. Max lives for the moment and has nothing holding him back. This unlikely couple are immediately attracted to each other.

They begin to find a deep mutual affection before disaster strikes. Suddenly rules and restrictions do not matter anymore. Doing the right thing is irrelevant. What matters most is that Max lives...

If you like your love and passion hinted at, rather than explicitly thrown in your face, then you will love this book.

Love in the Maldives – Naomi Davies

A holiday romance where no one is quite who they say they are! *The first novella in the Sixty Minute Romance Series*

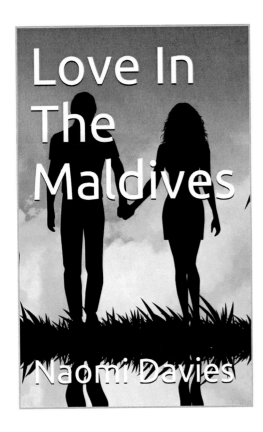

A romantic story set in the sunshine and the splendour of a Maldivian island. A holiday romance where no one is quite who they say they are. Follow the flight from London to the magnificent holiday island that Sandra and her best friend Anne take. This tropical paradise was made for romance.

Description from back cover of the print edition.

Sandra Wrighton was having a bad year. This included breaking up with her boyfriend after catching him in bed with someone else, and losing her job. Her solution was to go on a fabulous, all inclusive holiday to the Maldives with her best friend.

Even before she took the flight from Heathrow, she was hoping to meet a nice guy for some holiday romance and a bit of fun. The reality was far more unexpected and exhilarating.

For The Love of Music – Naomi Davies

A Romance Where Love Overcomes Appearances

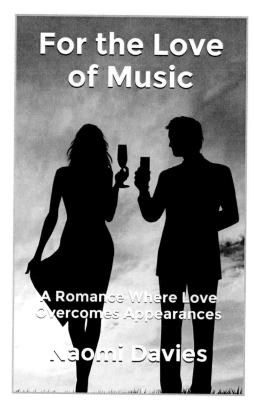

The Second Novella in the Sixty Minute Romance Series.

Anne Richardson was beautiful and alluring. She didn't even have to work at it. She always looked good. This tended to stop all but the bravest of men approaching her. Ed was that bravest of men.

But he was brash, unshaven, unkempt and with straggly uncut hair. More than that, he had been severely injured in Afghanistan and was now recovering from multiple wounds and a missing right leg. There is no way that these two people could fall in love, was there?

The Welsh Victorian Dolls Mystery – Naomi Davies

Where Love Blossoms in the Midst of Danger

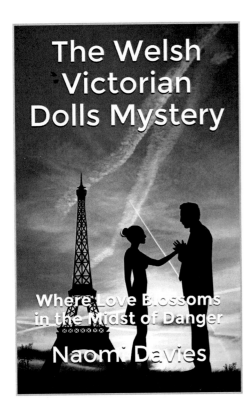

The Third Novella in the Sixty Minute Romance Series

Fiona Makin loved her little antique shop. It was in a sleepy English village and it was her whole life. There was no room, or time, for love in Fiona's life. She was far too busy. That was until she was saved from being run over by a car. Her rescuer was the mysterious William Ayres. He pretended to be interested in Victorian Welsh Dolls, but he wasn't. He was enigmatic, evasive and always in the midst of trouble. This quickly became a major problem for him, because he had fallen in love at first sight with Fiona. How could he win her heart over?

Look out for more romance titles from Naomi Davies coming soon.

Go to: **NaomiDavies.com**

Email: contact@naomidavies.com

Made in the USA
Middletown, DE
03 January 2018